Critical Care Focus

5: Antibiotic resistance and Infection Control

EDITOR
DR HELEN F GALLEY
Lecturer in Anaesthesia and Intensive Care
University of Aberdeen

EDITORIAL BOARD
PROFESSOR NIGEL R WEBSTER
Professor of Anaesthesia and Intensive Care
University of Aberdeen

DR PAUL G P LAWLER
Clinical Director of Intensive Care
South Cleveland Hospital

DR NEIL SONI
Consultant in Anaesthesia and Intensive Care
Chelsea and Westminster Hospital

DR MERVYN SINGER
Reader in Intensive Care
University College Hospital, London

© BMJ Books 2001
BMJ Books is an imprint of the BMJ Publishing Group

First published in 2001
by BMJ Books, BMA House, Tavistock Square,
London WC1H 9JR
Second impression 2001

www.bmjbooks.com
www.ics.ac.uk

British Library Cataloguing in Publication Data

A catalogue record for this book is available from the British Library

ISBN 0-7279-1538 X

The chapters in this book are based on presentations given at the Intensive Care Society's "It's a Bug's Life" Meeting, London, April 2000.

Typeset by FiSH Books Ltd.
Printed and bound by J W Arrowsmith Ltd., Bristol

Contents

Contributors

Julian F Bion
Reader in Intensive Care Medicine, University of Birmingham and Honorary Consultant in Intensive Care, University Hospital Birmingham NHS Trust.

Christian Brun-Buisson
Professor and Co-Director Medical Intensive Care Unit, and Director of the Infection Control Unit and Infection Diseases Teaching Programme, Hôpital Henri Mondor, Creteil, Paris.

Jean Chastre
Professor of Medicine, Hôpital Bichat, Paris.

Thomas SJ Elliott
Microbiologist, University Hospital Birmingham NHS Trust.

Vanya Gant
Consultant Microbiologist and Associate Clinical Director for Infection at the Hospital for Tropical Diseases, University College London Hospitals NHS Trust.

Lisa Glen
Department of Pharmacy, University Hospital Birmingham NHS Trust.

Ian M Gould
Consultant in Clinical Microbiology and Honorary Senior Lecturer, Aberdeen Royal Infirmary.

Hilary Humphreys
Professor of Microbiology, Royal College of Surgeons of Ireland and Consultant Microbiologist, Beaumont Hospital, Dublin.

Alan P Johnson
Clinical Scientist, Central Public Health Laboratory, London.

David M Livermore
Director, Antibiotic Resistance Monitoring and Reference Laboratory, Central Public Health Laboratory, and Honorary Senior Lecturer, St Bartholomew's and the Royal London School of Medicine and Dentistry.

Introduction

Infection on the intensive care unit: the scale of the problem

Julian F Bion, Thomas SJ Elliott, Lisa Glen

Infectious diseases are one of the commonest causes of death in the world, despite an ever-increasing range of antimicrobial agents. At the same time, in the developed world, large sums are expended on antimicrobial drugs with little evidence of efficacy, including their use in critically ill patients. Intensive care contributes only a small part to the world-wide use of antimicrobial agents, but it is an important element in the hospital economy. The use of these drugs should form part of an agreed hospital-wide strategy, based on collaborative practice, and must include an examination of the structure and processes of care, as well as monitoring outcomes. Simple measures are likely to be the most effective, and each intensive care unit should nominate a lead individual to facilitate infection control. This article examines the problem of infection and antimicrobials in terms of the intensive care unit population.

Infection control on the intensive care unit

Hilary Humphreys

When infection control strategies are successfully implemented in the intensive care unit, there is a significant "knock on" effect throughout the rest of the hospital as patients are regularly transferred to and from this area, often at short notice. It also reiterates the nature of intensive care, which is unpredictable, with staff often working under considerable pressure. This has implications for infection control, in particular the devising and implementation of strategies to minimise risk. Compliance of healthcare staff with basic infection control protocols such as hand washing regimens is generally poor, and staff shortages lead to difficulties in compliance with isolation precautions. The successful implementation of guidelines for optimising antibiotic use and slowing the emergence of antibiotic resistance, requires a multidisciplinary approach including managers, clinicians, general and specialist nurses, infectious diseases specialists, infection control teams, microbiologists and pharmacists. Despite the fact that infection control guidelines are based more on expert opinion than on the results of randomised controlled trials in many instances, it is clear that effective solutions to antibiotic resistance should be geared to the specific local epidemiological circumstances, and the available facilities and resources.

Colonisation or infection?

Jean Chastre

The definition of colonisation is the presence of micro-organisms, which, in contrast to infection, result in no overt detrimental clinical symptoms. This article will focus on respiratory tract colonisation and infection, and three key issues will be discussed. Firstly, the concept that colonisation of patients on the intensive care unit with micro-organisms is inevitable. Secondly, with the first premise in mind, the issue of whether antimicrobial treatment of colonised patients should be undertaken, and finally, the use of routine microbiological surveillance procedures for detecting infecting micro-organisms in intensive care unit patients.

Catheter-related infection

Christian Brun-Buisson

Despite the potential for prevention, catheter related infections still impose a substantial burden on critically ill patients, accounting for up to 25% of nosocomial infections. Prevention strategies include maximal barrier precautions during insertion, strict asepsis during manipulation and avoidance of systematic changes of both catheters and dressings. Continual surveillance and audit is essential to provide up to date protocol. This review describes how new measures now available such as tunnelling of catheters and the use of antibiotic or antiseptic impregnated devices may be particularly useful when infections rates remain high despite best intentions.

Mechanisms of antibiotic resistance

Alan P Johnson, David M Livermore

Antibiotics kill sensitive bacteria, but resistant ones survive. Thus, the intense selection pressure generated by antibiotic usage is such that resistance to many widely used antibiotics has increased alarmingly. There is no easy solution to the problem posed by resistance but it is likely that reduction and optimisation of antibiotic use is the way forward, backed by more rapid and accurate microbiology, development of new antibiotics, and protection of existing antibiotics from resistance determinants.

Knowledge of the local epidemiology of infection and resistance patterns is critical, together with knowledge of the likelihood of particular antibiotics to select resistance. It is not clear why some strains or genes spread widely whereas others, although equally resistant, do not. The relative importance of these sources of accumulated resistance varies according to the bacterial species but it should be remembered that all these processes are driven by the selective pressure of antibiotic use.

Antibiotic rotation to control resistance

Ian M Gould

Patients admitted to intensive care units are at greater risk of hospital acquired infection than other hospitalised patients. Antibiotic resistant organisms are more difficult and costly to treat such that limitations have to some extent been placed upon the ability to treat some bacterial infections. It has been suggested that rotation or cycling through different classes of antibiotic may reduce the incidence of resistant organisms. It is almost certain that there is a causative association between antibiotic use and the development of resistance. Given the recent world-wide escalation in resistance and the overwhelming evidence of unnecessary antibiotic use, the sensible approach to the control of antibiotic resistance is to control antibiotic use. The important question is how, rather than whether, but much research is still needed. It is probably the case that limiting antibiotic prescribing and not conscious antibiotic cycling is the way forward. This article reviews the evidence for limitation of bacterial resistance using such antibiotic rotation strategies.

Antibiotic policies in the intensive care unit

Vanya Gant

All antibiotics alter normal bacterial flora, and antibiotic resistant strains are selected, resulting in cross infection and colonisation. Resistance to antibiotics compromises therapy, and policies or guidelines for antibiotic prescribing may help to rationalise and reduce antibiotic usage, resulting in a reduction in costs and delaying the emergence of resistance. This article addresses issues relating to proscriptive antibiotic policies on the intensive care unit. The approach to limitation of emergence of resistance should be multi faceted: through reduced and more appropriate antibiotic prescribing and adequate infection control. Combinations or high dose regimens for existing antibiotic should be used where possible, and effective agents should be restricted to multi resistance infections. Most importantly the doctors prescribing should be educated to the dangers of antibiotic over- and inappropriate-use.

1: Infection on the intensive care unit: the scale of the problem

JULIAN F BION, THOMAS SJ ELLIOTT, LISA GLEN

Introduction

Infectious diseases are one of the commonest causes of death in the world, despite an ever-increasing range of antimicrobial agents. In the 1998 World Health Organisation (WHO) report on leading causes of death world-wide, infection was the second commonest cause of death after cardiovascular disease (Figure 1.1). In 1998, 13.3 million people died from infectious causes (25% of all deaths), equivalent to 25 people dying of infection every minute.[1] Most importantly, 50% of deaths occur in children under the age

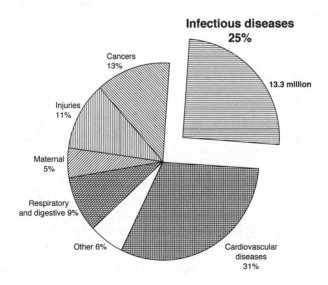

Figure 1.1 Leading causes of death world-wide in 1998. There were 53.9 million deaths from all causes. Note cancers, cardiovascular and respiratory/digestive deaths can also be caused by infections and raise the percentage of deaths to infection even further. Reproduced with permission from Ferlay J, Parkin DM, Pisani P. Cancer incidence and mortality worldwide. Geneva: World Health Organisation, 1998.

of five years, and four million children die from diarrhoeal disease each year. As predisposing factors, nearly one billion people are severely malnourished; every few seconds, someone in the world dies of starvation. At the same time in the developed world large sums are expended on antimicrobial drugs with little evidence of efficacy, including their use in critically ill patients. This article will examine the problem of infection and antimicrobials in terms of the intensive care unit (ICU) population.

Emergence of resistance: general aspects

In 1990, the WHO reported that in Thailand, where there is already substantial resistance of malaria to chloroquine and sulphodoxine pyrimethamine, 45% of malarial parasites were also resistant to quinine and mefloquine. In Japan, 60% of all staphylococci were multi-drug resistant; in Portugal 13% of *Mycobacterium tuberculosis* were resistant to single therapy and 4% were resistant to multidrug therapy.[2] International travel has increased markedly over the last 50 years (Figure 1.2), and will contribute to the spread of antimicrobial resistance. Prescribing controls vary widely between countries; in many, potent antibiotics are available to any with the resources to buy them. Even in those countries with strict prescribing controls in the community, antimicrobial resistance is becoming a common phenomenon in hospital practice and in ICUs.

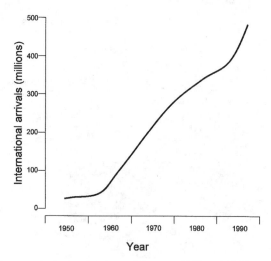

Figure 1.2 Increases in international travel between 1950 and 1990, paralleling the spread in antibiotic resistance.

It is not just human usage of antibiotics that causes the emergence of resistance. Antibiotics are also used indiscriminately in farming as growth promoters. Up to 80% of all livestock entering the food chain are exposed to antibiotics. In the USA alone, over 8500 tons of antibiotics are used each year in animal husbandry.

Infections in the ICU: epidemiology

The ICU is a particularly important focus for studying the epidemiology of infection. In 1992, a point prevalence survey[3] of infection in European ICUs was conducted. This important study involving 10 038 patients receiving treatment in 1417 ICUs in 17 countries, demonstrated that on the day of the study, 45% of patients were infected, and 21% had acquired their infections in the ICU. Another 10% had nosocomial (hospital-acquired) infection, while 14% had become infected in the community before admission to hospital. The most common organism identified was the gram-positive bacterium *Staphylococcus aureus*. The most common site of infection overall was the respiratory tract; nosocomial pneumonia is a particular concern given the potential adverse effects on survival.[4,5]

Mortality related to infection rates in European ICUs has also been studied.[3] At the time of the EPIC study, methicillin-resistant *S. aureus* (MRSA) was very common in countries such as France, Spain, Portugal and Italy, whilst the UK had a relatively low incidence, and this accounts for some of the variation presented in Figure 1.3. The apparently low infection rate in the UK in relation to overall mortality is surprising given

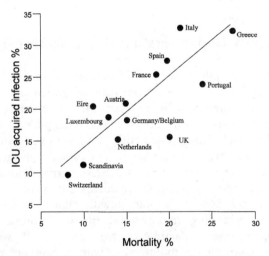

Figure 1.3 The relationship between the incidence of ICU-acquired infections and mortality in European intensive care units. Reproduced with permission from Vincent JL, Bihari DJ, Suter PM, et al. The prevalence of nosocomial infection in intensive care units in Europe. Results of the European Prevalence of Infection in Intensive Care (EPIC) Study. EPIC International Advisory Committee. Reproduced with permission from J Am Med Assoc 1995;274:639–44.

the overall high levels of severity of illness for UK ICU patients,[6] and it would be interesting to examine the hypothesis that reduced infections could be a consequence of the high nurse:patient ratio provided as a standard in UK ICUs.[7, 8]

In the USA, the National Nosocomial Infections Surveillance System reported data on 181 993 ICU patients for the 5-year period from 1992 to 1997, and showed that urinary tract infections were amongst the most common type of infection (31%) and infection was clearly linked to the use of urinary catheters.[9] Pneumonia was related to mechanical ventilation, with a predominance of gram-negative infections and bacteraemia was related to central venous and pulmonary artery catheterisation, with a preponderance of gram-positive organisms. There was considerable variation in infection rates between ICUs participating in the study, but no apparent relationship with ICU size or overall length of stay – more detailed measures of case mix are not available.

The incidence of bacteraemia over a 25-year period has been reported.[10] A mixture of organisms was responsible, including *Staphylococcus* and *Pseudomonas*, with a more recent trend towards an increase in bacteraemia rates and the identification of cephalosporin-resistant *Pseudomonas*. This was attributed to increased use of this class of antimicrobial agent, and greater frequency of use of central venous catheters (CVCs). These findings demonstrate the potential for harm associated with instrumentation and antibiotic prescribing and emphasises the importance of reviewing the methods used for the insertion and care of CVCs and the prescription of antibiotics.

Why do critically ill patients develop infections?

The high incidence of infection in ICU patients is related in part to increased susceptibility to infection from disease, patient and treatment factors (Box 1.1); however, it is also an inevitable consequence of concentrating the most severely ill and usually infected patients in one area of the hospital. Although these patients may not have been admitted with an infection, they may well already have been exposed to antimicrobial agents in the hospital or community, and therefore arrive with a modified flora of their own, containing resistant organisms. Intensive care does not exist in isolation, and close collaboration with clinical microbiology is important in understanding the hospital microenvironment and in implementing appropriate infection control policies. Preventing the progression from colonisation to infection with potentially pathogenic micro-organisms in an individual patient requires a "systems approach" involving multidisciplinary care throughout the institution.

Infection may be acquired from exogenous or endogenous sources. Both are important in critically ill patients, and it is of the utmost importance that all staff recognise their individual responsibility for minimising transmission of organisms from their own hands and clothing. The main endogenous sources are the patient's skin and gastrointestinal tract. Retrograde spread of organisms from bowel to oropharynx to lungs in the intubated patient is well recognised, but it has become a sufficiently common phenomenon for staff to accept it as a "normal" consequence of critical illness.

Box 1.1 Factors affecting susceptibility of critically ill patients to infection

- Bacterial translocation
- Instrumentation – endotracheal tubes, intravascular cannulae, urinary catheters
- Patient position
- Antimicrobial treatment
- Staff
- Immunological competence
- Nutritional depletion
- Genetic factors

Of current interest are genetic determinants of susceptibility to infection. A clinical study investigating survival status and cause of death amongst adult adoptees and their biological parents has demonstrated a five-fold increased risk of death if one of the natural parents had died from infection,[11] demonstrating the impact of genetic rather than environmental factors in determining the response to infection. Gene-related differences have been identified as important for many other infectious diseases (Table 1.1), though studied in greatest detail for malaria.[12] Other studies have implicated gene-related differences in cytokine responses to infection as a cause for differences in survival from critical illness, but the data are at present conflicting.[13,14] The majority are a consequence of genetic polymorphisms rather than whole gene defects, and as there are likely to be in the region of 100 000 possible polymorphisms in the human genome, the range of possible interactions between gene effects and the environment is huge and therefore difficult to predict.

In addition to the more obvious invasive interventions which may promote infection, other causes should be considered. These include transfusion of non-leucocyte-depleted blood, a factor which could possibly explain the adverse effects of blood transfusion identified by the Canadian critical care collaborative study, which demonstrated a trend towards a higher mortality with a more liberal transfusion threshold.[15]

Table 1.1 Examples of genetic factors influencing susceptibility to infection

	Mediated by	Susceptibility
Malaria (vivax)	Duffy antigen −ve	↓
Malaria (falciparum)	SSHb, G6PD, α Thal	↓
Malaria	TNF, NOS2, ICAM1	↑
Leprosy	HLA variant DR2	↑
Tuberculosis	IFγr-1 mutation	↑
Salmonella	IL-12r β1 chain	↑
Meningococcus	TNF promoter	↑
Endotoxin	TLR-4 r gene	↓

Prevention of infection

Clinical detection

Our ability to detect and differentiate colonisation from infection is discussed in Chapter 3. Clinical methods, although important, have their limitations. An investigation[16] of 93 critically ill patients identified episodes of pyrexia in 70%, but only half of these were judged to have an infectious cause. Only those episodes of pyrexia lasting more than 5 days were significantly associated with mortality. Clinical assessment needs to be supplemented by microbiological information in conjunction with other laboratory tests such as, for example, procalcitonin.

Infection control and environmental monitoring

In 1846 Semmelweis conducted what was in effect a prospective controlled trial, in which he demonstrated that the mortality from puerperal sepsis could be reduced from 11.4% to 1.27% by banning concurrent attendance at post-mortem examinations by doctors and students, and introducing handwashing with chloride of lime. His findings were largely ignored, and he died in obscurity. The story is well known, but even now staff fail to comply effectively with hand disinfection. A video surveillance study in Japan (a country where personal hygiene is of considerable cultural importance) showed that although 94% of relatives of patients in an ICU complied with handwashing protocols, the rate amongst ICU staff was only 71%.[17] Preventing transmission of microbes by staff requires leadership by example, effective hand disinfection equipment at each bed space, education and audit, and adequate staffing numbers (Box 1.2).

Box 1.2 Strategies to limit nosocomial infection

- Staff hand disinfection
- Nursing patients in a semi-recumbent position
- Subglottic aspiration in intubated patients
- Reduced duration of instrumentation
- Selective digestive decontamination
- Antimicrobial prescribing policies
- Enteral nutrition

Body position

The use of a supine body position has been shown to increase the risk of nosocomial pneumonia in ventilated patients.[18] A comparison of supine versus semi-recumbent (45 degree head-up) body position revealed a marked difference in nosocomial pneumonia rates: 8% compared with 34% (P < 0.003). When nasogastric feeding was combined with the supine position, pneumonia rates rose to 54%. This simple and zero-cost manoeuvre of altering the position in which patients are nursed, should be adopted as routine, and ICUs could use this measure to audit the efficacy of their overall approach to infection control.

Instrumentation

The association between central venous catheters and bacteraemia is well recognised. There are several approaches to reduce the risk. The most obvious is to minimise the frequency and duration of insertion by regular clinical review. The second is to improve the way these catheters and their taps, injection ports and syringes are handled by staff, particularly when patients are managed outside the ICU (for example, in the operating theatre). Carelessness at the time of insertion in theatre may result in CVC-related bacteraemia several days later. The third is the development of catheters with antimicrobial properties, including those with an electrical charge.[19] Similar comments apply to the use of urinary catheters in terms of minimising the duration of insertion.

Selective decontamination of the digestive tract

Selective decontamination of the digestive tract (SDD) has been shown to reduce markedly the incidence of microbial colonisation and nosocomial pneumonia, and it also has a modest effect on mortality, as demonstrated in the meta-analysis by D'Amico et al.[20] Despite this, SDD is not widely used, perhaps because of concerns about possible adverse effects on the microbiological environment. SDD acts by preserving the normal enteric anaerobic flora and eradicating pathogenic gram-negative aerobes and fungi. Its primary effect is to prevent these pathogens from gaining access to the oropharynx and lungs by microaspiration – an effect which can also be achieved by the semi-recumbent posture at lower cost and with little effect on the microbial environment, though this comparison has yet to be performed. However, there may be a role for SDD when used selectively in high-risk groups to prevent translocation via other routes, or to limit translocation of endotoxin.

Antibiotic policies, cost containment and collaborative practice

It is difficult to prove that antibiotic-prescribing policies make a difference to outcomes, but it is likely that the absence of agreed practice guidelines is irrational, impedes education of trainees, and probably increases costs (see Chapter 7). Guidelines facilitate clinical practice, make it easier to audit, and can be very simple. The most important element is joint daily review of antimicrobial prescriptions by clinician, microbiologist, and pharmacist. Feedback of information about expenditure from pharmacy databases (Figure 1.4) needs to be combined with data on case mix for interpretation, but could help to focus attention on the potential for changing practice or reducing expenditure.

National approaches to infection control

Nosocomial infections affect nearly 10% of all hospital patients and cost the National Health Service some £1 billion per year, resulting in prolonged hospital stays. In 30% of cases infection could be prevented; if half of these were prevented, this would result in savings of around £150 million.[21] The National Audit Office has recommended that infection control becomes part of each hospital trust's strategic agenda, with ultimate responsibility resting with the chief executive. They also recommend written policies and procedures, greater compliance with handwashing, active research, education, training and audit. Infection control teams should be adopting a pro-active role with proper follow-up after hospital care of high-risk groups. There is now a national infection surveillance scheme with 140 participating hospitals, similar to the American National Nosocomial Infections Surveillance System.

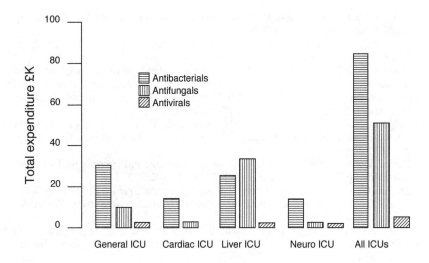

Figure 1.4 Six-month antimicrobial expenditure for four ICUs in one UK teaching hospital.

This should be combined with the appointment of nominated individuals in each ICU with responsibility for implementing infection control policies. Such policies must be developed with all participants in the care process, including domestic staff and management. Teaching, training and education must be multidisciplinary and, most importantly, infection control should form part of the undergraduate curriculum for all healthcare professionals in order to facilitate a cultural change in attitudes to infection prevention.

Conclusion

Intensive care contributes only a small part to the world-wide use of antimicrobial agents, but it is an important element in the hospital economy. The use of these drugs should form part of an agreed hospital-wide strategy, based on collaborative practice, and must include an examination of the structure and processes of care, as well as monitoring outcomes. Simple measures are likely to be the most effective, and each ICU should nominate a lead individual to facilitate infection control.

References

1 Ferlay J, Parkin DM, Pisani P. *Cancer incidence and mortality worldwide.* Geneva: World Health Organisation, 1998.
2 Dendoung S. *Malaria control programs in four different communities in Thailand.* Geneva: World Health Organisation, 1990.
3 Vincent JL, Bihari DJ, Suter PM, *et al.* The prevalence of nosocomial infection in intensive care units in Europe. Results of the European Prevalence of Infection in Intensive Care (EPIC) Study. EPIC International Advisory Committee. *J Am Med Assoc* 1995; **274**:639–44.
4 Kollef MH, Silver P, Murphy DM, Trovillion E. The effect of late-onset ventilator-associated pneumonia in determining patient mortality. *Chest* 1995; **108**:1655–70.
5 Torres A, Anzar R, Gatell JM, *et al.* Incidence, risk, and prognostic factors of nosocomial pneumonia. *Am Rev Resp Dis* 1990; **142**:523–8.
6 Le Gall JR, Lemeshow S, Saulnier F. A new Simplified Acute Physiology Score (SAPS II) based on a European/North American multicenter study. *J Am Med Assoc* 1993; **270**:2957–63.
7 Reis Miranda D, Ryan DW, Schaufeli WB, Fidler V, eds. *Organisation and management of intensive care. A prospective study in 12 European countries.* Berlin: Springer, 1997.
8 Department of Health. *Guidelines on admission to and discharge from intensive care and high dependency units.* London: NHS Executive, 1996.
9 Richards MJ, Edwards JR, Culver DH, Gaynes RP. Nosocomial infections in medical intensive care units in the United States. National Nosocomial Infections Surveillance. *Crit Care Med* 1999; **27**:887–92.
10 Edgeworth JD, Treacher DF, Eykyn SJ. A 25-year study of nosocomial bacteremia in an adult intensive care unit [see comments]. *Crit Care Med* 1999; **27**:1421–8.
11 Sorensen TI, Nielsen GG, Andersen PK, Teasdale TW. Genetic and environmental influences on premature death in adult adoptees. *New Engl J Med* 1988; **318**:727–32.
12 Kwiatkowski D. Genetic dissection of the molecular pathogenesis of severe infection. In: Bion JF, Brun-Buisson C, eds. Infection and critical illness: genetic and environmental aspects of susceptibility and resistance. *Intensive Care Med* 2000; **26(suppl)**:S89–97.
13 Westendorp RGJ, Langermans JAM, Huizinga TWJ, *et al.* Genetic influence on cytokine production and fatal meningococcal disease. *Lancet* 1997; **349**:170–3.
14 Stüber F, Petersen M, Bokelmann F, Schade U. A genomic polymorphism within the tumor necrosis factor locus influences plasma tumor necrosis factor-alpha concentrations and outcome of patients with severe sepsis. *Crit Care Med* 1996; **24**:381–4.
15 Hebert PC, Wells G, Blajchman MA, *et al.* A multicenter, randomized, controlled clinical trial of transfusion requirements in critical care. Transfusion Requirements in Critical Care Investigators, Canadian Critical Care Trials Group. *New Engl J Med* 1999; **340**:409–17.
16 Circiumaru B, Baldock G, Cohen J. A prospective study of fever in the intensive care unit. *Intensive Care Med* 1999; **25**:668–73.

17 Nishimura S, Kagehira M, Kono F, Nishimura M, Taenaka N. Handwashing before entering the intensive care unit: what we learned from continuous video-camera surveillance. *Am J Infect Control* 1999; **27**:367–9.

18 Drakulovic MB, Torres A, Bauer TT, *et al*. Supine body position as a risk factor for nosocomial pneumonia in mechanically ventilated patients: a randomised trial. *Lancet* 1999; **345**:1851.

19 Elliott T. Intravascular catheter-related sepsis — novel methods of prevention. In: Bion JF, Brun-Buisson C, eds. Infection and critical illness: genetic and environmental aspects of susceptibility and resistance. *Intensive Care Med* 2000; **26(suppl)**:S45–50.

20 D'Amico R, Pifferi S, Leonetti C, Torri V, Tinazzi A, Liberati A. Effectiveness of antibiotic prophylaxis in critically ill adult patients: systematic review of randomised controlled trials. *Br Med J* 1998; **316**:1275–85.

21 National Audit Office web site: http://www.nao.gov.uk/

2: Infection control on the intensive care unit

HILARY HUMPHREYS

Introduction

When infection control strategies are successfully implemented in the intensive care unit (ICU), there is a significant "knock on" effect throughout the rest of the hospital as patients are regularly transferred to and from this area, often at short notice. The results of a recent study examining the outcome in patients discharged from ICUs in the UK in the middle of the night compared to normal working hours emphasise the shortage of ICU beds,[1] necessitating untimely discharge practice. It also reiterates the nature of ICU care, which is unpredictable, with staff often working under considerable pressure. This has implications for infection control, in particular the devising and implementation of strategies to minimise risk.

Rise in antibiotic resistance

Over the last 20 years, gram-positive cocci have become the commonest pathogens causing hospital infections, mainly due to their capacity to develop antibiotic resistance.[2] The most obvious example is methicillin resistant *Staphylococcus aureus* (MRSA).[3] The prevalence of MRSA colonisation and infection are lower in countries with a more restrictive approach to antibiotic use, where infection control measures are rigorously enforced, and where nurse-to-patient ratios are higher. Infection control measures, including the routine use of gloves, gowns, hand antisepsis and the decolonisation of MRSA carriers, have met with varying degrees of success.[4] Most strains of MRSA are resistant to the majority of antibiotics, such that glycopeptides antibiotics, for example vancomycin, are the treatment of choice for systemic infection. Recently, there have been treatment failures in Japan and the USA caused by strains that were vancomycin intermediate methicillin-resistant *S. aureus* or VISA.[5,6] Where this occurs, there are few therapeutic options left, and the emergence of

VISA strains suggests that containment of MRSA transmission and restriction of vancomycin use in hospitals is essential.

Enterococci, which are part of the normal flora of the intestinal and genital tracts, are emerging as increasingly important hospital pathogens.[2,7] Inherent resistance to most commonly used antibiotics and the development of resistance to other agents by mutation or by transfer of resistance genes has contributed to this. Acquired vancomycin resistance has increased dramatically amongst enterococci in the USA from 0.3% in 1989 to 10% in 1995.[2] This increase has been mirrored by a large increase in the use of vancomycin. Many vancomycin-resistant strains are resistant to other antibiotics and the attributable mortality is substantial in those patients with bacteraemia due to these strains.[8] Although the incidence of infection caused by multiple-resistant enterococci remains lower in Europe than in the USA, outbreaks have been reported, particularly in transplant centres and ICUs.[9] As up to 5% of the population are intestinal carriers of vancomycin-resistant *Enterococci faecium*, according to one particular study,[10] there is a reservoir there which may spread and cause infection in the appropriate circumstances.

A gradual increase in multiple antibiotic resistance in a number of gram-negative hospital pathogens, notably *Klebsiella pneumoniae*, *Enterobacter* spp., *Pseudomonas aeruginosa* and *Acinetobacter* spp., has been observed. Intense antibiotic use in many hospitals, particularly ICUs, has preceded epidemic and endemic infections by these multiple resistant strains. A recent survey of European hospitals found that 23% of isolates of *Klebsiella* species were resistant to third-generation cephalosporins.[11] In many cases epidemic strains of these bacteria are resistant to almost all of the antibacterial drugs currently available, resulting in nosocomial pneumonia and bacteraemia, with an associated high mortality. The implementation of isolation strategies for colonised patients and the implementation of antibiotic policies to curtail inappropriate antibiotic prescribing are effective control measures.

Transmission of resistance on the ICU

The selection of resistant mutant strains from patients' own bacterial flora during antibiotic treatment, or the transfer between bacteria of mobile genetic determinants of resistance (such as plasmids and transposons – see Chapter 5), are the initiating steps in the development of resistance, followed by spread of resistant strains among patients in hospital. Among the critically ill patients in the ICU, selection of resistant bacteria is enhanced by the way in which patients are treated and the invasive procedures undertaken. The length of stay in the ICU or in the hospital, the duration and doses of broad-spectrum antibiotic treatment, the severity of underlying illness, the use of invasive devices such as intravenous catheters, and surgery, are all important risk factors for hospital-acquired or ICU-acquired infection, including that caused by antibiotic-resistant strains of bacteria. In addition, factors relating to patients themselves such as immune suppression, or the presence of a large bacterial inoculum as a reservoir of resistant mutants (e.g. a non-draining abscess), are also important. Other factors depend on the medical management; for example the use of monotherapy rather than combination therapy may favour selection of resistance in some infections; sub-optimum antibiotic doses or inappropriate routes of administration, such that bactericidal concentrations are not reached at the site of infection, also predispose to the emergence and spread of resistance.

When the endogenous microflora is altered during antibiotic treatment and replaced by resistant strains, patients are more likely to become colonised or infected with resistant flora. Commonly, transmission occurs as a result of contact between patients via the contaminated hands of doctors and nurses, or sometimes via inadequately decontaminated equipment. Outbreaks with a common source of multiple resistant bacteria, often caused by organisms such as *Pseudomonas* spp. and *Acinetobacter* spp., may be related to exposure of patients to contaminated equipment, or fluids; for example, during mechanical ventilation or endoscopy.

Standards for intensive care units

In a survey of 240 UK ICUs in 1992, it was reported that 14% of units had no isolation cubicles and less than 30% of beds were single rooms.[12] Guidelines on Standards for Intensive Care Units were issued by the Intensive Care Society (ICS) in 1997 and the European Society of Intensive Care Medicine (ESICM) in 1995.[13,14] Some issues are particularly germane to infection control and the most obvious perhaps is space. Recommendations were made for at least 20 m^2 floor space for each bed and at least one or two isolation cubicles in a ten-bedded unit, with wash handbasins for at least every other patient area. Many ICUs do not fulfil these recommendations and even if units were upgraded now, these recommendations could not be met without difficulty in many centres. Minimum air changes to provide adequate ventilation are also defined.

These issues are not just important for infection control, but also play a vital part in terms of the comfort of staff working in the ICUs. Often ICUs are extremely warm, stuffy and cluttered areas, and these conditions are not ideal considering the level of service of care provided. Frequent design errors include carpets in clinical areas, inaccessible sinks, and doors too narrow for moving equipment.[15]

Most clinicians will agree that isolation facilities are an essential component of the ICU, but the rationale as to which patients should be isolated, when, and for how long, is less clear. The isolation of an infected patient provides a physical barrier that can be important in preventing the spread of resistant organisms. But what is the evidence that isolation is of benefit? Much of the evidence, for example in the control of MRSA infections, is difficult to interpret since there are often multiple and simultaneous interventions undertaken during an outbreak, and consequently it is difficult to separate the efficacy of one intervention versus another. In a report from France in 1994,[16] conversion of an ICU from seven cubicles and two four-bedded rooms to 15 enclosed isolation rooms, resulted in a decrease in bronchopulmonary colonisation with *Acinetobacter* such that 12% of patients were colonised before the conversion compared to only 1% after. Clearly this report suggests that not only is the actual space itself important but the form and layout also.

Infection control strategies

Cleaning

In a study from Nottingham, sporadic infections with *Acinetobacter* spp., punctuated by prolonged outbreaks of infection involving larger numbers of patients caused by a particular epidemic strain of *Acinetobacter*, have occurred in an adult ICU since 1985.[17] Patients admitted to the ICU for three or more days during a non-outbreak period in 1994–95 were screened for the epidemic strain and DNA fingerprinting techniques were used to compare isolates of *Acinetobacter* with isolates obtained from the same ICU during the previous 10 years. Almost 20% of the ICU patients screened during 1994–95 became colonised with *Acinetobacter*. Environmental sampling yielded *Acinetobacter* from one or more samples on four occasions. Therefore the long-term persistence of a potentially epidemic strain in the ICU, even during a non-outbreak period, indicates a need for continued vigilance with regards to environmental decontamination for this and other nosocomial pathogens.

ESICM recommends that specialised cleaning personnel should be available to the ICU, who are familiar with infection prevention protocols and the hazards of medical equipment.[14] This is not always achievable, however, due predominantly to shortages of staff.

Hand washing

A significant proportion of medical staff do not always wash their hands when they should and its importance as an infection prevention measure is not appreciated widely enough. Transmission of micro-organisms from the hands of healthcare workers is the main cause of nosocomial infections, and handwashing remains *the* most important preventative measure.[18] Unfortunately, compliance with handwashing is unacceptably low in most institutions.[19]

A study reported in the *New England Journal of Medicine* eight years ago compared two different hand-washing regimens – chlorhexidine versus alcohol. The authors reported only around 40% compliance with either regimen despite an impressive on-going educational campaign.[20] What we wash our hands with is probably not as important as whether we wash our hands! In a University Hospital in Geneva, hand washing in 48 wards throughout the hospital was monitored by infection control nurses.[21] Compliance was 48% overall; the lowest compliance rate (36%) was found in ICUs, particularly before high-risk procedures (Table 2.1).

Table 2.1 Factors associated with non-compliance with hand washing. Reproduced with permission from Pittet D, Mourouga P, Perneger TV. Compliance with handwashing in a teaching hospital. *Ann Intern Med* 1999;**130**:126–30

Variable	Compliance (%)
Healthcare worker	
Nurse	52
Doctor	30
Nursing assistant	47
Other	48
Location	
Medical ward	52
Surgical ward	47
Intensive care unit	36

There is a mistaken belief that using gloves is an effective alternative to handwashing,[22] but failure to change contaminated gloves is at least as common as failure to wash hands.[18] Furthermore, removing gloves may contaminate hands and hence washing hands after glove use is important. Non-compliance with hand washing is a substantial problem and interventions aimed at improving hand-washing practices may be more effective if they focus on selected wards, specific groups of healthcare workers or certain patient care situations. The relationship between high workload and poor compliance suggests that over-concentrating on maximising staff productivity may conflict with high standards of patient care. A feasible approach is to minimise the time spent hand washing by providing alcohol hand rubs by patients' beds.[21] This is also a realistic solution to the situation where there are insufficient wash handbasins or they are too far away to use regularly.

Nursing staff levels

Staffing on the ICU is an important issue for infection control. Both the ICS and the ESICM suggest a 1 : 1 nurse : patient ratio for intensive care and 1 : 2 (ICS) or 1 : 3 (ESICM) for high-dependency care.[13,14] But what is the evidence that inadequate levels contribute to infection in the ICU? In 1996, an outbreak of central venous catheter (CVC) related bacteraemia was studied, focusing particularly on an outbreak of bacteraemia in the ICU. The results showed that nursing hours worked were less and patient : nurse ratios higher during the bacteraemia outbreak,[23] such that the more patients who were looked after by one nurse, the more likely the patient was to develop CVC bacteremia. In another study, from a neonatal ICU, a cluster of cases of *Enterobacter cloacae* was associated with the absence of several nurses.[24]

Conclusions

Compliance of healthcare staff with basic infection control protocols such as hand-washing regimens is generally poor, and staff shortages lead to difficulties in compliance with isolation precautions. The successful implementation of guidelines for optimising antibiotic use and slowing the emergence of antibiotic resistance, requires a multidisciplinary approach including managers, clinicians, general and specialist nurses, infectious diseases specialists, infection control teams, microbiologists and pharmacists (see Chapter 7). Despite the fact that infection control guidelines are based more on expert opinion than on the results of randomised controlled trials in many instances, it is clear that effective solutions to antibiotic resistance should be geared to the specific local epidemiological circumstances, and the available facilities and resources.

References

1 Goldfrad C, Rowan K. Consequences of discharges from intensive care at night. *Lancet* 2000; **355**:1138–42.
2 Gold HS, Moellering RC. Antimicrobial-drug resistance. *N Engl J Med* 1996; **335**:1445–3.
3 Voss A, Milatovic D, Wallrauch-Schwarz C, Rosdahl VT, Braveny I. Methicillin-resistant *Staphylococcus aureus* in Europe. *Eur J Clin Microbiol Infect Dis* 1994; **13**:50–5.
4 Mulligan ME, Murray-Leisure KA, Ribner BS, *et al.* Methicillin-resistant *Staphylococcus aureus*: a consensus review of the microbiology, pathogenesis, and epidemiology with implications for prevention and management. *Am J Med* 1993; **94**:313–28.

5 Hiramatsu K, Aritaka N, Hanaki H, et al. Dissemination in Japanese hospitals of strains of *Staphylococcus aureus* heterogeneously resistant to vancomycin. *Lancet* 1997; **350**:1670–3.

6 CDC Update. *Staphylococcus aureus* with reduced susceptibility to vancomycin. United States 1997. *MMWR* 1997; **46**:813.

7 Frieden TR, Munsiff SS, Low De, *et al.* Emergence of vancomycin-resistant enterococci in New York City. *Lancet* 1993; **342**:76–9.

8 Shay DK, Maloney SA, Montecalvo M, *et al.* Epidemiology and mortality risk of vancomycin-resistant enterococcal bloodstream infections. *J Infect Dis* 1995; **172**:993–1000.

9 Jordens JZ, Bates J, Griffiths DT. Faecal carriage and nosocomial spread of vancomycin-resistant *Enterococcus faecium*. *J Antimicrob Chemother* 1994; **34**:515–28.

10 Endtz HP, Van den Braak N, Van Belkum A, et al. Fecal carriage of vancomycin-resistant enterococci in hospitalized patients and those living in the community in the Netherlands. *J Clin Microbiol* 1997; **35**:3026–31.

11 Livermore DM, Yuan M. Antibiotic resistance and production of extended-spectrum ß-lactamases amongst *Klebsiella* spp. from intensive care units in Europe. *J Antimicrob Chemother* 1996; **38**:409–24.

12 Inglis TJ, Sprout LJ, Hawkey PM, Knappett P. Infection control in intensive care units: UK national survey. *Br J Anaesth* 1992; **68**:216–20.

13 Intensive Care Society. *Standards for intensive care units*. Intensive Care Society, London, 1997.

14 European Society of Intensive Care Medicine. *Minimal requirements for intensive care departments. Recommendations of the European Society of Intensive Care Medicine Task Force.* European Society of Intensive Care Medicine, Brussels, 1995.

15 Carter CD, Barr BA. Infection control issues in construction and renovation. *Infect Control Hosp Epidemiol* 1997; **18**:587–96.

16 Mulin B, Rouget C, Clement C, *et al.* Association of private isolation rooms with ventilator associated *Acinetobacter baumannii* pneumonia in a surgical intensive care unit. *Infect Control Hosp Epidemiol* 1997; **18**:499–503.

17 Webster CA, Crowe M, Humphreys H, Towner KJ. Surveillance of an adult intensive care unit for long term persistence of a multiresistant strain of *Acinetobacter baumannii*. *Eur J Clin Microbiol Infect Dis* 1998; **17**:171–6.

18 Larson EL. APIC guideline for handwashing and hand antisepsis in health care settings. *Am J Infect Control* 1995; **23**:251–69.

19 Jarvis WR. Handwashing – the Semmelweiss lesson forgotten? *Lancet* 1994; **344**:1311–12.

20 Doebbeling BN, Stanley GL, Sheetz CT, *et al.* Comparative efficacy of alternate hand washing agents in reducing nosocomial infection in intensive care units. *N Engl J Med* 1992; **327**:88–93.

21 Pittet D, Mourouga P, Perneger TV. Compliance with handwashing in a teaching hospital. *Ann Intern Med* 1999; **130**:126–30.

22 Doebbeling BN, Pfaller MA, Houston AK, Wenzel RP. Removal of nosocomial pathogens from the contaminated glove. Implications for glove re-use and handwashing. *Ann Intern Med* 1988; **109**:394–8.

23 Fridkin SK, Pear SM, Williamson TH, Galgiani JN, Jarvis WR. The role of understaffing in central venous catheter associated bloodstream infections. *Infect Control Hosp Epidemiol* 1996; **17**:150–8.

24 Harbroath S, Sudre P, Dharan S, Cadenas M, Pittet D. Outbreak of *Enterobacter cloacae* related to understaffing, overcrowding and poor hygiene practices. *Infect Control Hosp Epidemiol* 1999; **20**:598–603.

3: Colonisation or infection?

JEAN CHASTRE

Introduction

The definition of colonisation is the presence of micro-organisms, which, in contrast to infection, result in no overt detrimental clinical symptoms. This article will focus on respiratory tract colonisation and infection, and three key issues will be discussed. Firstly, the concept that colonisation of patients on the intensive care unit (ICU) with micro-organisms is inevitable, secondly, with the first premise in mind, the issue of whether antimicrobial treatment of colonised patients be undertaken, and finally, the use of routine microbiological surveillance procedures for detecting infecting micro-organisms in ICU patients.

Is colonisation inevitable?

As we have known for many years and clearly demonstrated by many studies, it is practically impossible to avoid tracheal colonisation in mechanically ventilated patients in the ICU.[1-3] For example, one study of a large series of ICU patients showed that nearly 90% of patients were colonised with gram-negative *Enterobacteriaceae*.[4] Most of the micro-organisms were *Pseudomonas aeruginosa* and exactly the same results have been consistently documented in several subsequent studies. Clearly, avoiding colonisation in intubated patients in the ICU is going to be very difficult. Prevalence of colonising bacteria in ICU patients is directly related to the duration of mechanical ventilation, which was nicely demonstrated in a study by A'Court *et al.* in 1994.[2] Using invasive techniques to directly assess distal airway colonisation, these authors could demonstrate that, after 10 days and 20 days of mechanical ventilation, 5% and 14% of patients, respectively, had evidence of distal colonisation. However, after 30 days of mechanical ventilation nearly 35% were colonised. Obviously distal airway colonisation is not present during the first day of mechanical ventilation and only becomes evident after a longer period of ventilation.

In a study from Barcelona, 48 ICU patients with medical and/or surgical head injury were investigated.[3] The colonisation rate was measured at different times at various sites – the nasal site, at the pharyngeal site and also in the trachea and, using bronchoscopy, at the distal site. The study showed that even only a few hours after the injury, at the beginning of mechanical ventilation, nearly 50% of the patients were colonised by group 1 micro-organisms including *Streptococcus pneumoniae*, methicillin-susceptible *Staphylococcus aureus* (MSSA) and *Haemophilus influenzae*. This pattern of colonisation persisted until the 10th day of mechanical ventilation. Although the rate of group 2 organisms (particularly *Enterobacteriaceae*, *Pseudomonas aeruginosa* and *Acinetobacter*) was very low initially, after 5 or 6 days of mechanical ventilation, nearly 50% of the patients were colonised by these micro-organisms. Not only was the rate of patients colonised by group 2 and group 1 micro-organisms high, but the bacterial burden presented into the trachea was also very high: after 10 days' mechanical ventilation, the mean sum of colony forming units was 10^{10} per ml respiratory secretions, which is a very high bacterial burden.

In the same study, it was shown that the development of early-onset ventilator-associated pneumonia was clearly related to the presence or absence of tracheal colonisation with group 1 micro-organisms. In patients not colonised by group 1 micro-organisms the rate of nosocomial pneumonia was very low (<10%), but it was >50% in patients who were colonised with group 1 micro-organisms after 6 days of mechanical ventilation.[3] By contrast, risk factors directly associated with late-onset ventilator-associated pneumonia were tracheal or bronchial colonisation with group 2 micro-organisms (odds ratio 5.4), duration of prior mechanical ventilation (odds ratio 7.7) and, very interestingly, prolonged antibiotic treatment after initiation of mechanical ventilation (odds ratio 11).[3]

Is prophylactic antibiotic treatment useful?

Prophylactic antibiotics used to try to suppress tracheal colonisation with endogenous flora results in a high rate of ventilator-associated pneumonia and most regimes have little or no effect on mortality rates.[5] In addition, prophylactic antibiotics promote emergence of multidrug-resistant micro-organisms. A study by Johanson *et al* published in 1988 investigated mechanically ventilated baboons treated with a variety of regimens of intravenous and topical antibiotics, or no antibiotics at all.[1] In the absence of antibiotics, pneumonia occurred in almost all animals and was polymicrobial. However, in baboons which were receiving prophylactic topical polymycin, the incidence of pneumonia was only slightly decreased and the prevalence of drug-resistant micro-organisms in the tracheal secretions was very high: 60% after 4 days of mechanical ventilation and 78% after 8 days of mechanical ventilation, respectively.[1] This study suggests that the prophylactic use of antibiotics in the ICU increases the risk of infection with multi-resistant pathogens, while only delaying the occurrence of nosocomial infection.

Probably a much more useful strategy in the ICU would be to try to avoid the use of broad-spectrum antibiotics. This was nicely demonstrated by de Man in a very recent paper in the *Lancet*.[6] In this study, the authors investigated whether the emergence of resistant strains could be halted by modifying the empirical antibiotic regimens to remove the selective pressure which favours resistant bacteria. Two identical neonatal ICUs were assigned to different empirical antibiotic regimens. On unit A, penicillin G and tobramycin were used for early-onset septicaemia, flucloxacillin and tobramycin were used for late-onset septicaemia, but no broad-spectrum beta-lactam antibiotics, such as amoxicillin and cefotaxime, were used. In unit B, intravenous amoxicillin with cefotaxime was the empirical therapy. After 6 months of the study the units exchanged regimens. Rectal and respiratory cultures were taken on a weekly basis. There were 436 admissions, divided equally between the two regimens (218 in each). Three neonates treated with the penicillin–tobramycin regimen became colonised with bacilli resistant to the empirical therapy used, versus 41 neonates on the amoxicillin–cefotaxime regimen ($P < 0.0001$). The relative risk for colonisation with strains resistant to the empirical therapy per 1000 at-risk patient days was 18 times higher for the amoxicillin–cefotaxime regimen compared with the penicillin–tobramycin regimen. *Enterobacter cloacae* was the predominant bacillus in neonates on the amoxicillin–cefotaxime regimen, whereas *Escherichia coli* predominated in neonates on the penicillin–tobramycin regimen. These colonisation patterns were also seen when the units exchanged regimens.[6] Therefore, policies addressing the empirical use of antibiotics do matter in the control of antimicrobial resistance. A regimen avoiding amoxicillin and cefotaxime may restrict such resistance problems.

There are some potential advantages of using antibiotics prophylactically for eradicating endogenous micro-organisms once colonisation has occurred. Firstly, eradicating such micro-organisms may reduce the rate of subsequent infection. Secondly, it may also be possible to reduce the chance that the micro-organisms will be transmitted from colonised patients to other susceptible patients in the same ICU. However, there are also some potential shortcomings of such a policy. Fagon and co-workers recently reported the results of a large, prospective, randomised trial comparing non-invasive versus invasive diagnostic management of 413 patients suspected of having ventilator-associated pneumonia (VAP).[7] In the non-invasive group ($n = 209$), empirical antimicrobial therapy was

based on the presence of bacteria in the gram stain of endotracheal aspirates, and therapy could be adjusted or discontinued according to the results of semiquantitative cultures. In the case of severe sepsis, empirical therapy was started without the laboratory result. With this schedule, which resembles clinical practice in most ICUs, 91% of patients (191/209) received empirical therapy for suspected VAP and only 7% did not. The invasive work-up ($n = 204$) consisted of bronchoscopy with direct microscopic examination, and empirical therapy was started only if results were positive. A definitive diagnosis based on quantitative culture results of specimens obtained with a protected specimen brush or by bronchoalveolar lavage was awaited before starting, adjusting or discontinuing therapy. The strategy resulted in treatment in 52% of patients (107/204) with VAP, whereas 44% (90/204) did not receive antibiotics.[7] In addition, compared with patients who received clinical management, patients who received invasive management had reduced mortality at day 14 (16% and 25%; $P = 0.022$), decreased mean sepsis-related organ failure assessment (SOFA) scores at day 3 (6 ± 4 and 7 ± 4, respectively, $P = 0.033$) and at day 7 (5 ± 4 and 6 ± 4 respectively, $P = 0.043$). Antibiotic use was also decreased (mean number of antibiotic-free days, 5 ± 5 and 2 ± 3 days respectively, $P < 0.001$). At 28 days, the invasive management group had significantly more antibiotic-free days (11 ± 9 compared with 7 ± 7 days, $P < 0.001$). Multivariate analysis showed a significant difference in mortality (hazard ratio, 1.54 [CI, 1.10 to 2.16], $P = 0.01$) (Figure 3.1).

Thus, implementation of bronchoscopic techniques in the diagnosis of ventilator-associated mortality reduces antibiotic use and improves outcome for patients.[7] The study also provides answers to common concerns held. Is it safe to withhold antibiotics if microscopic examination of bronchoscopy samples is negative? Yes, since empirical antibiotics were withheld in 97 of 114 patients (85%) and only seven received antibiotics after quantitative culture results became available. Is it safe to guide empirical therapy on the results of direct microscopic examination? Yes, since only one patient in the invasive group received initial inappropriate empirical therapy, compared with 24 of 191 patients in the non-invasive group, even though 22 of the latter had been treated according to recommended guidelines. Are cases of VAP missed because the sensitivity of invasive techniques may not be 100%? Hardly, since there were only three new cases of pneumonia in the first 3 days after randomisation in this group. By contrast, there were 22 infections at other sites requiring specific therapeutic measures in the invasive group and only five in the non-invasive group. This difference suggests that reliance on non-invasive techniques and the consequent overestimation of VAP may mean that diagnoses of non-pulmonary infections get missed.

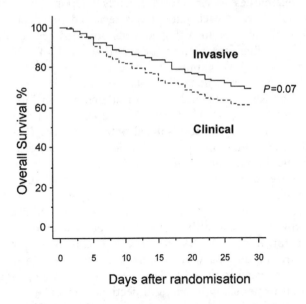

Figure 3.1 Actual mortality in a large, prospective, randomised trial comparing non-invasive (clinical) versus invasive diagnostic management of 413 patients suspected of having ventilator associated pneumonia. See text for details of study design. Reproduced with permission from Fagon JY, Chastre J, Wolff M, et al. Invasive and noninvasive strategies for management of suspected ventilator-assisted pneumonia. Ann Intern Med 2000;132:621–30.

Are routine surveillance procedures useful?

The issue of whether routine surveillance cultures are useful in the prediction of infecting micro-organisms in the ICU has been addressed by several investigators.[8–10] In theory, cultures may predict patients with invasive disease and may assist in determining initial treatment. However two studies published three decades ago by Evans *et al.* demonstrate disappointing results.[8,9] The ability of routine surveillance cultures to predict sepsis in a very large study of neonates in the ICU was only 60%, whilst specificity was only 80%, with a positive findings predictive value for the routine surveillance cultures of only 7.5%. Clearly this was not a very good result.

Culture results from routine microbiological specimens obtained prior to the onset of VAP in ICU patients may help to predict the causative micro-organisms of lung infection and thus the selection of effective empirical antimicrobial therapy. A prospective study of 125 consecutive episodes of VAP in which the causative micro-organisms were determined using bronchoscopic techniques was reported recently.[11] Upon entry into the study, the hospital chart of each patient was reviewed prospectively and culture results of all microbiological specimens obtained previously were recorded (mean number per patient, 38 ± 39). A total of 220 micro-organisms were cultured at significant concentrations (protected brush specimens $>10^3$ cfu/ml, broncheoalevolar lavage specimens $>10^4$ cfu/ml) from bronchoscopic specimens and were considered responsible for lung infection. Seventy-one (57%) of the 125 episodes of VAP were polymicrobial. The most frequently isolated organisms were *P. aeruginosa* and other non-fermenting gram-negative bacilli (31%), *Enterobacteriaceae* (14%), and methicillin-resistant *S. aureus* (16%). Of these 220 organisms, only 73 (33%) were recovered prior to the onset of pneumonia (53 from pulmonary secretion cultures, 17 from systematic surveillance cultures, 21 from catheter tip cultures, 7 from blood cultures, and 8 from urine cultures) such that their susceptibility patterns were available for guiding empirical treatment. In only 40 (39%) of the 102 patients in whom prior culture results from pulmonary secretions were obtained (mean delay before the onset of pneumonia 8 ± 8 days) were all the micro-organisms ultimately found responsible for lung infection previously recovered. Furthermore, 372 organisms that were not responsible for VAP were also previously isolated, making prospective predictions of the true pathogens difficult. Based on these data, the role of routine microbiological specimens in guiding management decisions in patients with suspected VAP appears limited.[11]

Conclusion

In summary, it seems to be impossible to avoid tracheal colonisation in most patients receiving mechanical ventilation in the ICU. Secondly, using antibiotics prophylactically for preventing infection in these patients without evidence of infection is a major way of selecting for the emergence of resistant micro-organisms, although in a minority there may be a role for preventing transfer of colonising organisms between patients. The benefit of routine surveillance cultures has not been demonstrated.

References

1 Johanson WG Jr, Seidenfeld JJ, de los Santos R, Coalson JJ, Gomez P. Prevention of nosocomial pneumonia using topical and parenteral antimicrobial agents. *Am Rev Respir Dis* 1988; **137**:265–72.

2 A'Court CH, Garrard CS, Crook D, *et al*. Microbiological lung surveillance in mechanically ventilated patients, using non-directed bronchial lavage and quantitative culture. *Q J Med* 1993; **86**:635–48.

3 Ewig S, Torres A, El-Ebiary M, *et al.* Bacterial colonization patterns in mechanically ventilated patients with traumatic and medical head injury. Incidence, risk factors, and association with ventilator-associated pneumonia. *Am J Respir Crit Care Med* 1999; **159**:188–98.

4 Johanson WG Jr, Seidenfeld JJ, Gomez P, de los Santos R, Coalson JJ. Bacteriologic diagnosis of nosocomial pneumonia following prolonged mechanical ventilation. *Am Rev Respir Dis* 1988; **137**:259–64.

5 Bonten MJ, Kullberg BJ, van Dalen R, *et al.* Selective digestive decontamination in patients in intensive care. *J Antimicrob Chemother* 2000;**46**:351–62.

6 de Man P, Verhoeven BA, Verbrugh HA, Vos MC, van den Anker JN. An antibiotic policy to prevent emergence of resistant bacilli. *Lancet* 2000; **355**:973–8.

7 Fagon JY, Chastre J, Wolff M, *et al.* Invasive and non-invasive strategies for management of suspected ventilator-associated pneumonia. A randomized trial. *Ann Intern Med* 2000; **132**:621–30.

8 Evans HE, Akpata SO, Baki A. Factors influencing the establishment of the neonatal bacterial flora. II. The role of environmental factors. *Arch Environ Health* 1970; **21**:643–8.

9 Evans HE, Akpata SO, Baki A. Factors influencing the establishment of the neonatal bacterial flora. I. The role of host factors. *Arch Environ Health* 1970; **21**:514–19.

10 Finelli L, Livengood JR, Saiman L. Surveillance of pharyngeal colonization: detection and control of serious bacterial illness in low birth weight infants. *Pediatr Infect Dis J* 1994; **13**:854–9.

11 Hayon J, Chastre J, Trouillet JL. Role of serial routine microbiologic culture results in the initial management of ventilator-associated pneumonia. *Am J Respir Crit Care Med* 1998;**157**:A168(abstract).

4: Catheter-related infection

CHRISTIAN BRUN-BUISSON

Introduction

Despite their potential preventability, catheter-related infections still impose a substantial burden on critically ill patients. These infections account for about 20–25% of all nosocomial infections in intensive care unit (ICU) patients, including the so-called primary bacteraemias which account for about 50% of all nosocomial bacteraemias in the ICU. The estimated mortality attributable to catheter-related infection is about 10–15% and the excess length of stay 7–10 days. Most early catheter-related infections – i.e. within 30 days – and therefore most ICU-acquired catheter infections, are associated with colonisation at the skin entry site and subsequent infection along the subcutaneous tract of the catheter, whereas those occurring later may be more often associated with infection of the catheter hub during manipulations. This article will address the incidence and prevention of catheter-related infection in ICU patients.

Incidence of catheter-related infection

In hospitalised patients, central venous catheters are used frequently, particularly in patients in the ICU. Catheter-related infections account for a large percentage of nosocomial infections. Depending on which study and subspeciality is referred to, the incidence varies between 0.3 and 36 infectious episodes per 1000 catheter days. In general in a mixed medical, surgical and trauma ICU, the average incidence is five bacteraemic episodes per 1000 catheter days. To put the figures into perspective it has been reported that about 50 000 patients develop catheter-related sepsis each year in the USA,[1] and that in 1994 the deaths from catheter-related infections in Australia were more than the number of deaths from the acquired immunodeficiency syndrome.[2] The manifestations of catheter-related infection may range from locally restricted inflammation to life-threatening sepsis. The probability of catheter-related sepsis is suggested to be between 0.3 and 0.5% per day for the duration of catheterisation.[3] The vast majority of these infections are due to coagulase-negative staphylococci. These organisms were more common in central line-associated primary blood stream infections than in non-central line associated-infections.[4] Despite the number of deaths from catheter-related infection, compliance with written guidelines for central venous catheters' insertion technique and site care remains low.[5] Lack of compliance independently increases the risk of catheter-related infection fivefold,[6] whilst changing nurse : patient ratios from 1 : 1 to 1 : 2 increases risk by more than 60 times.[7]

Diagnosis of catheter-related infection

Diagnosing catheter-related infection without removing the catheter poses a problem. The diagnosis of catheter infection means a decision as to whether a febrile episode is definitely or possibly related to catheter infection and this will usually mean a positive result for blood culture and catheter tip culture or improvement of symptoms on catheter removal. When rapid information about catheter infection is needed, a gram stain can be obtained on the intravascular segment of the catheter, and this will correlate with culture techniques reasonably well. Obviously this requires catheter removal, and it also implies that any other primary infection is categorically excluded, which may be quite difficult.

Although a catheter may be suspected of being infected, in fact this is the case in only about 25% of instances, meaning that many catheters are removed unnecessarily. The predictive value of several markers of infection were studied by Armstrong in 1990.[8] Clinical symptoms such as erythema and pyrexia, and skin site and blood cultures were investigated. It was shown that skin site cultures showing more than 50 cfu were high predictors of infection, and erythema and temperature had relatively low predictive values.

Paired quantitative blood cultures have been proposed to establish the diagnosis of catheter-related infection without removing the catheter. A central-to-peripheral blood culture colony count ratio of between 5/1 and 10/1 is considered to be indicative of catheter-related infection, and this technique has been validated for long-term and short-term catheter placement.[9] However, this method is cumbersome, time consuming and expensive, and therefore not widely used in routine clinical practice. Measurement of the differential time to positivity between catheter hub-blood and peripheral-blood cultures may be an attractive alternative to quantitative blood cultures. A prospective study suggested that this technique is a simple and reliable tool for *in situ* diagnosis of catheter-related sepsis in cancer patients. However, further studies are needed to confirm these data for short-term catheters.[10]

Prevention of catheter-related infection

Bacterial colonisation increases dramatically with duration of catheterisation. There are several ways by which catheter infection can occur, but the two most common and important are colonisation of the catheter hub with intraluminal migration of pathogens into the bloodstream, and secondly, extraluminal migration of pathogens from the bloodstream from colonisation of the catheter insertion site. Several prospective studies have used molecular typing to characterise isolates which caused catheter-related bloodstream infections. In these studies, many bloodstream isolates were the same as those found on the skin insertion site and on catheter hubs.[11-13] These data suggest that preventative measures should aim to target both the insertion site and the catheter hub. One of the most important preventative measures is prevention of catheter colonisation during insertion, which can be achieved by using "maximal sterile barrier precaution" during insertion.[14] Tunnelling of the catheters should reduce extraluminal migration of bacteria into the bloodstream (see below).

Choice of site

There are a number of strategies which can be used to minimise catheter-related risk factors and perhaps the most obvious one is to limit the numbers of patients receiving central venous catheterisation. Select, if possible, a site that is at lower risk of infection such as subclavian instead of internal jugular or femoral sites. The bacterial bio-burden on the skin of the lower chest is less than that at the neck or femoral sites. However, there is a greater risk of mechanical complications at the subclavian site and this must be balanced against the suggestion that catheter-related infection risk is increased. Irrespective of the choice of site, many catheters become colonised at the time of insertion.[15]

Precautions during insertion

The choice of antiseptic used to clean the skin at the insertion site is an important component in preventing catheter-related infection. It has been shown that alcoholic chlorhexidine is more effective compared to povidone iodine.[16] It is important, however, that the alcohol is allowed to dry on the skin before the catheter is inserted, and this may take up to two or three minutes. Strict aseptic technique including large sterile drapes, and wearing of sterile gown, gloves, mask and cap, should also be strictly adhered to.[14]

Tunnelling of catheters

Tunnelling of catheters under the skin has been suggested to reduce catheter-related infection, particularly from those placed in the jugular vein, although a meta-analysis of seven studies concluded that there was no advantage to tunnelling of catheters for short-term use.[17] Another study found that the decreased incidence of catheter-related sepsis when catheters were tunnelled disappeared when a newly appointed catheter care nurse arrived in one ICU.[18]

Changing catheters

Scheduled changes of central venous catheters at fixed intervals are of no benefit, and may actually increase the infection risk, compared to as-needed replacement.[19] Replacement of central venous catheters can be achieved using placement of a new catheter at a new site or by using the Seldinger technique to change the catheter over a guidewire. This can be useful when a potentially infected catheter needs to be replaced in a febrile patient with no signs of infection at the catheter insertion site and no other obvious source of infection, and to avoid venepuncture in patients with poor venous access due to burns, obesity, or a coagulopathy. Studies have suggested that exchanging catheters over a guidewire may be associated with fewer mechanical complications, and no significantly increased risk of infection compared with placement of a new catheter at a different site, although this may to some extent reflect staff inexperience. A comprehensive review of the guidewire exchange strategy has suggested that although this technique may be associated with a somewhat increased catheter-related infection risk, there are fewer mechanical complications.[19] The US Hospital Infection Control Practices Advisory Committee supports new-site replacements and removal of the infected catheter in patients with documented catheter infection. However, the Committee recommends guidewire-assisted catheter exchange for either a malfunctioning catheter (with no evidence of infection at the catheter site) or when catheter-related infection is suspected but there is no purulence or erythema at the site. The offending catheter should be cultured and a new site subsequently accessed if the culture is positive.[1]

Choice of dressing and catheter material

The choice of dressing and indeed catheter material may have some bearing on the risk of catheter-related infection. An early meta-analysis suggested that the risk of catheter-related infection was increased by the use of transparent rather than gauze dressings.[20] However, newer highly permeable materials for transparent dressings may actually reduce infection rates,[21] and such dressings are now preferred to allow regular inspection of the insertion site for evidence of infection, without the need for replacing the dressing. Similarly to catheters, dressings need not be replaced at fixed intervals, and can be replaced as needed. Many approaches have been taken to improve catheter design to reduce the risk of catheter-related infection. Improvements in the shape of the catheter tips and re-engineering of the needle to aid non-traumatic skin penetration have been made. The use of a hydrophilic coating has been shown to reduce colonisation *in vitro*. Bacteria adhere differently to different catheter surfaces and the relationship of catheter material to infection risk is under investigation.

Antiseptic and antibiotic-coated catheters

A range of antimicrobial agents have been used to coat catheters in an attempt to reduce catheter-related sepsis; these include both antibiotics (used to treat patients) and antiseptics (used for skin preparation). Although catheters coated with teicoplanin prevented abscess formation in mice, in patients undergoing major abdominal surgery, the teicoplanin was only retained on the catheter for 36 hours and hence had no effect on catheter colonisation.[22] Minocycline and tetracycline have also been used to coat catheters. In a randomised double-blind controlled trial these catheters were shown to reduce microbial colonisation and decrease bacteraemia. Another trial of minocycline/rifampicin-coated catheters versus antiseptic-coated catheters showed less risk of colonisation and bloodstream infection when antibiotic was used.[23]

Coating catheters with antibiotics used to treat patients with infections has raised concern about the development of resistance. The use of topically applied antibiotic agents does lead to the emergence of resistance, although there is no evidence of resistance to the antibiotic used for catheter coating. However, the concern about resistance has lead in part to the development of antiseptic-coated catheters. Catheters which had been coated with iodine mixed with polyvinyl pyrrolidone or silver had less colonisation *in vitro* but have yet to be evaluated clinically. Other agents used include chlorhexidine gluconate with silver sulphadiazine coated onto the external surface of the catheter, shown in clinical use to reduce the incidence of bacteraemia by 60%,[24] although subsequent studies did not uphold these findings.[25] However, a meta-analysis of the use of these catheters in patients at high risk of catheter-related infection did report that both colonisation and infection were reduced.[26] In this latter study the aggregate risk reduction was about 50% in terms of both catheter colonisation and also incidence of catheter-related bacteraemia. Triple lumen catheters coated on both the internal and external surfaces with benzalkonium chloride have recently been developed. Although both *in vitro* and *in vivo* studies have shown reduced colonisation, further clinical studies are awaited. These antiseptic catheters only retain activity for about two weeks and therefore are most suited for short-term catheter use in higher risk patients.

Another novel approach which used low voltage electric current applied to carbon-impregnated colonised catheters revealed a potent bactericidal effect as a result of hydrogen peroxide and free chlorine release by electrolysis at the catheter surface. *In vitro* studies have also shown that silver iontophoretic catheters prevent colonisation with *Staphylococcus aureus*. Both of these techniques may provide a future method of preventing bacterial colonisation of catheters but clinical studies are awaited.

Conclusion

Many studies have been conducted in recent years and have greatly increased our understanding and ability to prevent catheter infection. More randomised controlled trials of, for example, different venous sites, multiple lumen versus single lumen catheters, the insertion technique, dressing type and frequency of change, skin cleansing regimens, and antiseptic and antibiotic coating of catheters, are required. The results of such studies should then enable improvement of the available clinical guidelines for the prevention and management of catheter-related infections.

References

1 Pearson ML for the Hospital Infection Control Practices Advisory Committee. Guideline for the prevention of intravascular device related infections. *Infect Control Hosp Epidemiol* 1996; **17**:438–73.
2 Collignon PJ. Intravascular associated sepsis: a common problem. *Med J Aust* 1994; **161**:374–8.
3 Eyer S, Brummitt C, Crossley K, *et al.* Catheter related sepsis: prospective, randomized study of three methods of long term catheter maintenance. *Crit Care Med* 1990; **18**:1073–9.
4 Richards MJ, Edwards JR, Culver DH, Gaynes RP and National Nosocomial Infections Surveillance System. Nosocomial infections in medical intensive care units in the United States. *Crit Care Med* 1999; **27**:887–92.
5 Roach H, Larson E, Barlett DB. Intravascular site care. Are critical care nurses practicing according to written protocols? *Heart Lung* 1996; **25**:401–8.
6 Ena J, Cercenado E, Martinez D, *et al.* Cross sectional epidemiology of phlebitis and catheter related infections. *Infect Control Hosp Epidemiol* 1992; **13**:15–20.
7 Fridkin SK, Pear SM, Williamson TH, *et al.* The role of understaffing in central venous catheter associated bloodstream infections. *Infect Control Hosp Epidemiol* 1996; **17**:150–8.

8 Quilici N, Audibert G, Conroy MC, *et al*. Differential quantitative blood cultures in the diagnosis of catheter-related sepsis in intensive care units. *Clin Infect Dis* 1997; **25**:1066–70.

9 Armstrong CW, Mayhall CG, Miller KB, *et al*. Clinical predictors of infection of central venous catheters used for total parenteral nutrition. *Infect Control Hosp Epidemiol* 1990; **11**:71–8.

10 Blot F, Nitenberg G, Chachaty E, *et al*. Diagnosis of catheter-related bacteraemia: a prospective comparison of the time to positivity of hub-blood versus peripheral-blood cultures. *Lancet* 1999; **354**:1071–7.

11 Mermel LA, McCormick RD, Springman SR, *et al*. The pathogenesis and epidemiology of catheter related infection with pulmonary artery Swan Ganz catheters. *Am J Med* 1991; **91**(suppl):197S–205S.

12 Maki DG, Stolz SS, Wheeler S, *et al*. A prospective randomized trial of gauze and two polyurethane dressings for site care of pulmonary artery catheters. *Crit Care Med* 1994; **22**:1729–37.

13 Maki DG, Stolz S, Wheeler S, *et al*. Prevention of central venous catheter related blood stream infection by use of an antiseptic-impregnated catheter. *Ann Intern Med* 1997; **127**:257–66.

14 Raad II, Hohn DC, Gilbreath J, *et al*. Prevention of central venous catheter-related infection by using maximal sterile barrier precautions during insertion. *Infect Control Hosp Epidemiol* 1994; **15**:231–8.

15 Elliott TSJ, Moss HA, Tebbs SE, *et al*. Novel approach to investigate a source of microbial contamination of central venous catheters. *Eur J Clin Microbiol Infect Dis* 1997; **16**:210–13.

16 Maki DG, Ringer M, Alvarado CJ. Prospective randomized trial of povidone iodine, alcohol and chlorhexidine for the prevention of infections associated with central venous and arterial catheters. *Lancet* 1991; **338**:339–43.

17 Randolph AG, Cook DJ, Gonzales CA, *et al*. Tunneling short term catheters to prevent catheter related infection: a meta analysis of randomized controlled trials. *Crit Care Med* 1998; **26**:1452–60.

18 Keohane P, Attrill H, Northover J, *et al*. Effect of catheter tunnelling and a nutrition nurse on catheter sepsis during parenteral nutrition. *Lancet* 1983; **ii**:1388–90.

19 Cook D, Randolph A, Kernerman P, Cupido C, King D, Soukup C, Brun-Buisson C. Central venous catheter replacement strategies: a systematic review of the literature. *Crit Care Med* 1997; **25**:1417–24.

20 Hoffman KK, Wever DJ, Samsa GP, Rutala WA. Transparent polyurethane film and an intravenous catheter dressing: a meta analysis of the infection risks. *J Am Med Assoc* 1992; **267**:2072–6.

21 Reynolds MG, Tebbs SE, Elliott TSJ. Do dressings with increased permeability reduce the incidence of central venous catheter related sepsis? *Intensive Crit Care Nurs* 1997; **13**:26–9.

22 Bach A, Darby D, Bottiger B, Bohrer H, Motsch J, Martin E. Retention of the antibiotic teicoplanin on a hydromer-coated central venous catheter to prevent bacterial colonization in post operative surgical patients. *Intensive Care Med* 1996; **22**:1066–9.

23 Darouriche RO, Raad II, Heard SO, *et al*. A comparison of two antimicrobial impregnated central venous catheters. *N Engl J Med* 1999; **340**:1–8.

24 Clemence MA, Jernigan JA, Titus MA, Duani DK, Farr BM. A study of antiseptic impregnated central venous catheters for prevention of bloodstream infections. In: *Program and Abstracts of the 33rd Interscience Conference on Antimicrobial Chemotherapy, New Orleans, LA*. Washington DC: American Society for Microbiology, abstract 1624, p 416.

25 Pemberton LB, Ross V, Cuddy P, Kremmer H, Fessler T, McGurk E. No difference in catheter sepsis between standard and antiseptic central venous catheters. *Arch Surg* 1996; **131**:986–9.

26 Veenstra DL, Saint S, Saha S, Lumley T, Sullivan SD. Efficacy of antiseptic impregnated central venous catheters in preventing catheter related bloodstream infections. *J Am Med Assoc* 1999; **281**:261–7.

5: Mechanisms of antibiotic resistance

ALAN P JOHNSON AND DAVID M LIVERMORE

Introduction

Antibiotics kill sensitive bacteria, but resistant ones survive. Thus, the intense selection pressure generated by antibiotic usage is such that resistance to many widely used antibiotics has increased alarmingly. For example, fifty years ago, the overwhelming majority of *Staphylococcus aureus* were sensitive to penicillin but nowadays 95% are resistant, due to production of ß-lactamase. Furthermore, although methicillin and other semi-synthetic penicillins not susceptible to hydrolysis by staphylococcal ß-lactamase were introduced in the 1960s, methicillin-resistant *S. aureus* (MRSA) subsequently emerged, now accounting for ≃40% of *S. aureus* from bacteraemias in the UK.[1] Until 1986, vancomycin was universally active against gram-positive cocci but now ≃25% of *Enterococcus faecium* are resistant in the UK, as are a smaller proportion of *E. faecalis* isolates.[1] World-wide, there are also reports of intermediate vancomycin resistance in a few MRSA isolates.[2] Third-generation cephalosporins were considered a panacea against gram-negative opportunists in the 1980s; today 30–40% of *Enterobacter* isolates are resistant.[3] Extended-spectrum ß-lactamases (ESBLs), enzymes that are able to hydrolyse most cephalosporins, have spread to around 25% of klebsiellae in European intensive care units (ICUs), also undermining the third-generation cephalosporins.[4] The carbapenems (imipenem and meropenem) have retained activity against most enterobacteria including those resistant to the cephalosporins but resistance has been increasingly noted in *Pseudomonas aeruginosa* and *Acinetobacter baumannii*.[5]

There is no easy solution to the problem posed by resistance but it is likely that reduction and optimisation of antibiotic use is the way forward, backed by more rapid and accurate microbiology, development of new antibiotics, and protection of existing antibiotics from resistance determinants. Knowledge of the local epidemiology of infection and resistance patterns is critical, together with knowledge of the likelihood of particular antibiotics to select resistance.

How are bacteria resistant?

There are several mechanisms that can confer bacterial resistance to antibiotics:

1   Production of enzymes that inactivate or modify the antibiotic (e.g. ß-lactamases, aminoglycoside-modifying enzymes, chloramphenicol acetyltransferase).
2   Modification of the drug's target site to reduce antibiotic binding (e.g. penicillin-binding proteins with reduced affinity for ß-lactams in pneumococci), or acquisition of a supplementary enzyme that by passes the antibiotic's target site (as applies in MRSA).
3   Reduced intracellular drug accumulation owing to reduced uptake (e.g. due to lack of specific outer membrane channels called porins) or to increased efflux of antibiotics from the bacterial cytoplasm or cytoplasmic membrane.

How do bacteria become resistant and how does resistance spread?

Mutation

Resistance in previously sensitive species can arise through mutations, which can be defined as random and spontaneous genetic changes. Antibiotics do not cause mutations to occur, but their use clearly generates an intense pressure for the selection of resistant mutants that arise naturally at low frequency. This selection of natural variants may be regarded as an extreme form of Darwinian evolution. The short generation time for bacterial replication mean that this "survival of the fittest" may be manifest within the time period that a patient receives a course of antibiotic treatment.

The rapid emergence of mutational resistance can swiftly reduce the effectiveness of an antibiotic. Fluoroquinolones were originally active against MRSA, but staphylococci have an efflux pump and resistance arises if this is upregulated by mutation of a gene called norA.[6] Most MRSA are now resistant and ciprofloxacin therefore has limited efficacy against infections due to these strains. Another example of rapid mutational resistance is given by the "third-generation" cephalosporins cefotaxime and ceftazidime. Such drugs initially appeared active against Enterobacter, Citrobacter and Serratia spp., but their activity depends only upon a failure to induce the chromosomal AmpC type ß-lactamase of these species. This means that the cephalosporins select for mutants (termed "derepressed") that constitutively hyperproduce these ß-lactamases.[7] These mutants occur relatively frequently (one cell per million), and the risk of their selection, and consequent clinical treatment failure, is thought to be $\simeq 20\%$ during cephalosporin therapy of *Enterobacter* bacteraemia. Resistant mutants may also spread among patients leading to strain epidemics.

Transfer of genetic material

Bacteria can acquire genetic resistance determinants from other bacteria, either as plasmids (loops of non-chromosomal DNA) or as chromosomal inserts. Chromosomal inserts include transposons – which are "sticky ended" sections of DNA able to "jump" from one DNA molecule to another – and genes transferred by bacteriophages (viruses that can infect bacteria). A few species, principally *Neisseria* spp., *Haemophilus* spp. and *Streptococcus pneumoniae*, can also absorb and incorporate fragments of DNA released from dead cells of related species. These fragments then combine with existing genetic material to form "mosaic" genes. This mechanism is the basis of penicillin resistance in pneumococci and pathogenic *Neisseria* spp.[8]

Gene epidemics

Plasmids and some chromosomally inserted transposons are often freely transmissible and their epidemic spread allows resistance to extend to diverse organisms. Plasmids encoding the TEM-1 type ß-lactamase were first noted in 1965 in *Escherichia coli* and have since spread to 20–60% of *Enterobacteriaceae* isolates, to a few strains of *P. aeruginosa* and to 1–50 % of *Haemophilus influenzae* and *Neisseria gonorrhoeae*, depending on the country.[7,9] The spread of these enzymes has meant that penicillin treatment without ß-lactamase inhibitors is no longer effective in serious infections involving gram-negative bacteria.

Plasmids coding one of the first ESBLs recorded – TEM-3 – spread among *Klebsiella*, *Escherichia coli* and *Serratia* spp. in several hospitals in France between 1985 and 1987,[10] and a single plasmid coding another ESBL – TEM-26 – spread among multiple *Klebsiella* and *E. coli* strains in several hospitals around Chicago in the mid-1990s.[11] A few gene epidemics have also demonstrated spread between gram-positive and gram-negative bacteria: for example tetracycline resistance conferred by *tetM* now occurs in streptococci and staphylococci, *Ureoplasma ureolyticum* and *N. gonorrhoeae*.[12]

The extent of epidemic gene spread partly depends upon the ability of the particular genes to transfer among plasmids, some of which have broader host ranges than others. In addition, some resistance genes occur in integrons, which can be thought of as a natural recombination system. Integrons can, cleverly, accumulate several resistance genes behind a single promoter, with the result that genes encoding resistance to some antibiotics may persist in the absence of use of the corresponding agent.[13]

The factors that determine whether a mobile gene will spread widely remain incompletely understood. For example, the TEM-2 type ß-lactamase differs from TEM-1 by just one amino acid and confers similar resistance. There is no obvious reason why one enzyme should achieve a greater evolutionary success than another, but numerous surveys have found the TEM-1 enzyme to be much more prevalent than TEM-2.[7,9]

The extra burden of replicating additional DNA in the absence of selection pressure (i.e. antibiotic use) might be expected to suggest that plasmid spread should be self-limiting, but there is little evidence for this optimistic view point. Indeed, many plasmid-mediated resistances are very widespread and persist despite the long absence of selection pressure (e.g. streptomycin resistance in *Enterobacteriaceae*).[13] These observations argue that plasmid carriage exerts little real burden.

Selection of resistant species

Emergence of new resistance phenotypes in hitherto susceptible species – as with vancomycin-intermediate *S. aureus* or carbapenem-resistant *Acinetobacter* – are more obvious and immediately disturbing than changes in the relative importance of different opportunist pathogens. Nevertheless, by killing sensitive organisms, antibiotics also open ecological niches for other strains or species with greater resistance. An example is vaginal candidiasis during protracted antibiotic use. However, this effect on microbial ecology is a much more serious problem in ICU patients, when compromised immunity results in vulnerability to repeated opportunistic infections. Winning an antimicrobial battle against one pathogen exposes an opening for more resistant organisms, both in the individual patient and the entire patient group. As an example *A. baumannii* and *Stenotrophomonas maltophilia* are increasingly seen in many ICUs, often from patients who have received multiple previous antibiotics.[14,15] *A. baumannii* isolates are often resistant to all drugs except carbapenems, and *S. maltophilia* responds only to co-trimoxazole and ticarcillin/clavulanate. Their inherent resistance is a likely factor in the emergence of these once rare pathogens. In addition, *Enterobacter* and *Serratia* species are more capable of developing resistance to cephalosporins than *E. coli*, and their increasing role as opportunist nosocomial pathogens in the critically ill may reflect the heavy use of cephalosporins.[9]

Strain epidemics

Patient-to-patient transfer of resistant strains is another important factor in the increasing resistance problem. Although mosaic gene formation and bacteriophage-mediated transfer of resistance genes are rare genetic events, strains that initially acquire their resistance by these mechanisms may subsequently spread rapidly and widely among patients. Nosocomial spread of resistant infections occurs all too commonly and may be related to inadequate infection control measures (see Chapter 2). The rising proportion of MRSA among *S. aureus* bacteraemias in England and Wales is shown in Figure 5.1. Until 1993 the proportion was steady at 1–2 % but

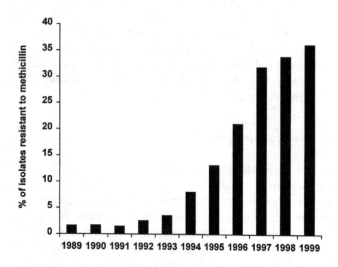

Figure 5.1 Rates of resistance to methicillin in Staphylococcus aureus *isolated from blood cultures.*

then rose steadily such that by 1998, the overall rate reached 36%.[1] This increase is thought to be attributable largely to the spread of two epidemic MRSA (EMRSA) strains, EMRSA15 and 16. The reasons for the epidemicity of these two strains is unclear as many equally resistant strains do not spread significantly. Both EMRSA15 and 16 strains are quinolone resistant and may have been advantaged by increasing use of these drugs. However, any *S. aureus* strain can readily become resistant to quinolone antibiotics, so it is difficult to believe that this is a complete explanation. The success of some multi-resistant *Klebsiella* strains is equally difficult to explain. In France a serotype K25 strain, which has SHV-4 type ß-lactamase, has spread widely, although this enzyme confers no greater resistance to third-generation cephalosporins than other ESBL types.[16] Intriguingly, the strain was among the first klebsiellae to become quinolone resistant,[17] and this may have helped its early spread. If this is the case its dominance may decline as quinolone resistance becomes more widespread among other strains.

The emergence of resistance continues to cause concern. Strategies include the developing new antibiotics, and prolonging the life of established antibiotics by, for example, combining with ß-lactamase inhibitors, or using antimicrobial drugs in combination. Clearly less, and more appropriate, use of antibiotics is required, as discussed elsewhere in this volume. The ecological and public health consequences of the use of antibiotics should never be overlooked.

Summary

Resistance can spread through species selection, mutation, gene epidemics, and strain epidemics. Current patterns of cephalosporin and quinolone use have ostensibly benefited some bacteria that are inherently resistant to these drugs. Mutational resistance may occur relatively frequently with some antibiotic/organism combinations, such that therapy may fail when resistant mutants are selected in individual patients. Escape of resistance genes to DNA capable of spreading to other bacteria (e.g. plasmids) is rare, but when it does occur, it allows the epidemic spread of resistance genes into different pathogens. Strain epidemics – the spread of strains of bacteria among patients – usually occur in individual units or hospitals and may reflect poor infection control. Particular strains achieve great success: for example much of the MRSA problem in the UK is due to the spread of two epidemic strains, EMRSA15 and 16. It is not clear why some strains or genes spread widely whereas others, although equally resistant, do not. The relative importance of these sources of accumulated resistance varies according to the bacterial species, but it should be remembered that all these processes are driven by the selective pressure of antibiotic use.

References

1 Reacher MH, Shah A, Livermore DM, *et al.* Bacteraemia and antibiotic resistance of its pathogens reported in England and Wales between 1990 and 1998: trend analysis. *Br Med J* 2000; **320**:213–16.
2 Johnson AP. Intermediate vancomycin resistance in *Staphylococcus aureus*: a major threat or a minor inconvenience. *J Antimicrob Chemother* 1998; **42**:289–91.
3 Livermore DM. ß-Lactamase-mediated resistance and opportunities for its control. *J Antimicrob Chemother* 1998; **41**(suppl D):25–41.
4 Babini G, Livermore DM. Antimicrobial resistance among *Klebsiella* spp. collected from intensive care units in Southern and Western Europe in 1997–1998. *J Antimicrob Chemother* 2000; **45**:1833–89.
5 Livermore DM, Johnson AP. Problems with resistant gram-negative bacteria: how to tackle them? *Drugs & Bugs* 2000; **6**:1–4.
6 Piddock LJ. Mechanisms of resistance to fluoroquinolones: state-of-the-art 1992–1994. *Drugs* 1995; **49**(suppl 2): 29–35.

7 Livermore DM. ß-Lactamases in laboratory and clinical resistance. *Clin Microbiol Rev* 1995; **8**:557–84.

8 Dowson CG, Coffey TJ. ß-Lactam resistance mediated by changes in penicillin-binding proteins. In: Woodford N, Johnson AP, eds. *Molecular bacteriology: protocols and clinical applications.* Totowa, NJ: Humana Press, pp 537–53.

9 Sanders CC, Sanders WE. ß-Lactam resistance in gram-negative bacteria: global trends and clinical impact. *Clin Infect Dis* 1992; **15**:824–39.

10 Petit A, Gerbaud G, Sirot D, *et al.* Molecular epidemiology of TEM-3 (CTX-1) ß-lactamase. *Antimicrob Agents Chemother* 1990; **34**:219–24.

11 Schiappa DA, Hayden MK, Matushek MG, *et al.* Ceftazidime-resistant *Klebsiella pneumoniae* and *Escherichia coli* bloodstream infection: a case-control and molecular epidemiologic investigation. *J Infect Dis* 1996; **174**:529–36.

12 Roberts MC. Genetic mobility and distribution of tetracycline resistance determinants. *Ciba Found Symp* 1997; **207**:206–18.

13 Chiew Y-F, Yeo S-F, Hall LMC, Livermore DM. Can susceptibility to an antimicrobial be restored by halting its use? The case of streptomycin versus *Enterobacteriacae. J Antimicrob Chemother* 1998; **41**:247–51.

14 Humphreys H, Towner KJ. Impact of *Acinetobacter* spp. in intensive care units in Great Britain and Ireland. *J Hosp Infect* 1997; **37**:281–6.

15 Muder RR, Yu VL, Dummer JS, *et al.* Infections caused by *Pseudomonas maltophilia*: expanding clinical spectrum. *Arch Intern Med* 1987; **147**:1672–4.

16 Buré A, Legrand P, Arlet G, Jarlier V, Paul G, Philipon A. Dissemination in five French hospitals of *Klebsiella pneumoniae* serotype K25 harbouring a new transferable enzymatic resistance to third generation cephalosporins and aztreonam. *Eur J Clin Microbiol Infect Dis* 1988; **7**:780–2.

17 Yuan M, Aucken H, Hall LMC, *et al.* Epidemiological typing of *Klebsiella* with extended-spectrum ß-lactamases from European intensive care units. *J Antimicrob Chemother* 1998; **41**:527–39.

6: Antibiotic rotation to control resistance

IAN M GOULD

Introduction

Patients admitted to intensive care units (ICUs) are at greater risk of hospital-acquired infection than other hospitalised patients. Antibiotic-resistant organisms are more difficult and costly to treat, such that limitations have to some extent been placed upon the ability to treat some bacterial infections. It has been suggested that rotation or cycling through different classes of antibiotic may reduce the incidence of resistant organisms. This article will review the evidence for limitation of bacterial resistance using antibiotic rotation strategies.

What do we mean by resistance?

The term antibiotic resistance is used frequently but influences on resistance are rarely considered. The concept that resistance is also dependent on pharmacodynamics and clinical outcome is often ignored. For example a strain of *Escherichia coli* which produces ß-lactamase (an enzyme related to penicillinase which destroys benzyl penicillin and confers resistance to penicillin) is resistant to ampicillin. This means that although a patient with a chest infection caused by such a strain cannot be treated, such strains can easily be killed by ampicillin concentrations of around 2000 mg/l in the laboratory which may be clinically achievable in the urinary tract. Susceptibility to an antibiotic varies with bacterial species. Clinical resistance is a complex interaction between the infecting bacteria, the infection site, the distribution and concentration of antibiotic and the immune status of the patient (Box 6.1). The mechanisms encoding antibiotic resistance can be divided into four types: drug inactivation or modification, alteration in target site, bypass pathways, and decreased uptake (see Chapter 5).

Box 6.1 Factors contributing to the emergence of antibiotic resistance in the ICU.

- Severity of underlying illness
- Invasive procedures
- Immunocompetence
- Antibiotic usage
- Poor infection control practice
- Use of broad-spectrum antibiotics

Thus the dynamics of resistance can be defined simply as the interaction between the organism, the drug (antibiotic), the patient, and the environment (ICU) (Figure 6.1).

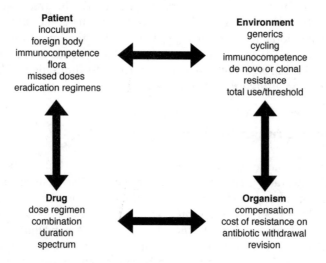

Patient
inoculum
foreign body
immunocompetence
flora
missed doses
eradication regimens

Environment
generics
cycling
immunocompetence
de novo or clonal
resistance
total use/threshold

Drug
dose regimen
combination
duration
spectrum

Organism
compensation
cost of resistance on
antibiotic withdrawal
revision

Figure 6.1 The interaction between the patient, the drugs prescribed, the organism and the environment in the development of antibiotic resistance. Reproduced with permission from Gould IM. A review of the role of antibiotic policies in the control of antibiotic resistance. J Antimicrob Chemother *1999;43:459–65.*

Genesis of antibiotic resistance on the ICU

Antibiotic resistance occurs as a direct consequence of antibiotic use.[1,2] An ICU provides an ideal location for the selection, maintenance and spread of antibiotic resistance in the hospital. An average ICU in a large teaching hospital will use about 10% of the antibiotic budget of the entire hospital, despite comprising only 1% of the total number of beds. This serves to illustrate the extent of antibiotic use and provides a tremendous selection pressure for bacteria to become resistant to multiple antibiotics. The problem of containing this level of resistance is now of major concern.

In individual patients there are several factors which can contribute to the development of resistance, such as a large inoculum, leading to increased potential for pre-existing resistant mutants, and any process which lowers drug concentrations at the site of infection. These circumstances tend to select out resistance, as will slower eradication of infection due to immunosuppression.[3] It is important to remember that although the normal bacterial flora are often ignored, treatment of infection inevitably also exposes normal flora to antibiotics. Development of resistance in normal flora may spread to more pathogenic organisms. Eradication of resistant pathogens by the use of selective digestive decontamination (SDD) regimens has proved disappointing, although eradication of colonising resistant organisms has occasionally been successful, particularly methicillin-resistant *Staphylococcus aureus* (MRSA).[4]

In terms of the patient, the genesis, maintenance and spread of antibiotic resistance is fostered by a number of circumstances particularly common to ICU patients. There has been concern about overprescribing of antibiotics for essentially as long as antibiotics have been on the market, and most doctors now accept that antibiotic resistance is a problem for everyone, and this problem is owned by most doctors because all doctors prescribe antibiotics. How this can be modified through altered prescribing habits is an area that is wide open for future research, and might include alteration in dose regimens, the use of combinations of antibiotics, rotation or cycling of different types of antibiotic class, or the length of the course of antibiotic.

Antibiotic rotation or cycling

It used to be thought that if the selection pressures for antibiotic resistance are lowered the organisms would revert to a sensitive form but we now know that that is clearly optimistic. Rapid removal of selection pressure may result in reversion to sensitivity, but this is likely to take longer than the original process of resistance. Resistant survivors may also undergo mutations over hundreds of generations to favour maintenance of the resistant gene. This seems to have happened for example with MRSA and vancomycin-resistant enterococci (VRE). Mathematical models suggest that compensation is more likely than reversion.[5]

The most complex situation is where multiple resistance mechanisms occur. The worst scenario is the presence of an integron, a type of transposon or sticky ended DNA which transfers from one genome to another, which can accommodate both resistant determinants and also the genes for their chromosomal integration and expression. This is explained in Chapter 5. Linked resistance is complex, as shown many years ago in bacteria which were dually resistant to both amoxicillin and trimethoprim, and where declining use of amoxicillin, even in the presence of increased trimethoprim use, led to a decline in trimethoprim resistance.[6] Resistance determinants coded for particular antibiotics on an integron will select for maintenance of resistance to all agents represented on that integron. Transposons can also code for active efflux of many different classes of antibiotics (the so-called "sump-pump" resistance mechanism). Although fluoroquinolones such as ciprofloxacin were initially effective against MRSA, it soon became clear that *Staphylococcus aureus* has an efflux system, effective against ciprofloxacin for example, but probably the primary role is for the rapid clearance of any foreign substance from biological membranes.[7]

The actual antibiotic is in itself important in the development of resistance. Narrow-spectrum agents in theory should have less effect on normal flora than broad-spectrum agents. In a previous review,[8] aminoglycosides particularly selected for resistance associated with a high incidence of treatment failure. The dosing schedule is also important. Higher doses, which result in higher drug concentrations at the site of infection, are less likely to select for resistance, although it is not known what repercussions this has on normal flora. In addition, combinations of antibiotics may be useful in preventing resistance.[8] Mathematical models favour combination therapy for preventing de-novo emergence of resistance.[9]

Containing resistance

In crucial areas like the ICU a direct relationship between the level of antibiotic use and resistance is seen, for example ceftazidime use and resistant *Enterobacter cloacae* and *Pseudomonas aeruginosa*, or MRSA and anti-staphylococcal penicillins and first-generation cephalosporins. The concept of using antibiotic rotation to control resistance (recently termed cycling) has re-emerged. There is some evidence of success, mostly concerning rotation of aminoglycosides, such as gentamicin and amikacin.[10] To prevent any resistant mutants becoming established, two-month periods of use have been proposed, although this cycling regimen may be rather frequent. Perhaps rotation on an individual-patient basis is just as practical, although this may not always be feasible. If possible, therapy should always be designed to give the least chance for selection of resistant strains. A cycling policy may also encourage the "unthinking" use of broad-spectrum antibiotics.

Several recent studies have shown the benefits of policies which reduce antibiotic use (both at a national level and also in individual hospitals) on resistance rates. In two large community-based studies in Iceland and Finland, there was a problem of penicillin-resistant pneumococci and erythromycin-resistant *Streptococcus pyogenes*. In Iceland[11] this followed the increased use of a wide range of antibiotics reaching a high of 23.2 defined daily doses (DDD)/1000 inhabitants/day in 1990, which was followed by a peak in penicillin resistance of 20% in 1992. By 1995, usage had decreased to 20.2 DDD/1000 inhabitants/day, mainly due to reduced penicillin resistance. Antibiotic use had been 15.5% during a 6-month period in 1992 and 9.2% in 1995. Resistance was particularly prevalent in young children in day-care centres, and was associated with clonal spread of a resistant strain (serotype 6B) from Spain. In Finland,[12] increased prescribing of erythromycin to treat Group A streptococcal throat and skin infections, resulted in increased erythromycin resistance (5% in 1988 to 19% in 1993). A subsequent 50% reduction in erythromycin use then led to resistance rates falling to 8.6% in 1996. This seems to be an example of a "critical threshold" being reached, in that resistance rates declined without total removal of the antibiotic, probably by reduced selection allowing suppressed, sensitive strains to become more dominant.

Recent studies in France[13,14] have shown reduced prevalence of gentamicin-resistant MRSA when gentamicin prescribing was decreased, and it has been suggested that decreasing vancomycin use may be beneficial in controlling VRE. In Greece, an 80% reduction in quinolone use was associated with decreased resistance rates amongst various gram-negative bacilli.[14] In another study, implementation of specific management protocols in an ICU cut antibiotic use by 50% and trends in terms of reduced resistance were seen.[14] Other studies have shown that altered antibiotic-prescribing habits substantially reduced the use of broad-spectrum agents with significant decreases in the rates of nosocomial bacteraemia, selected gram-negative bacteraemia, MRSA colonisation or infection, and *Stenotrophomonas maltophilia* colonisation or infection.[14] These decreases could not be attributed to changes in patient demographics or infection control practices.

In response to an outbreak of multiresistant *Acinetobacter* sp. infection, which was not controlled by infection control procedures, a restrictive antibiotic policy was introduced in an ICU in the USA, such that approval was needed for certain antibiotics including amikacin, aztreonam, ceftazidime, imipenem, ciprofloxacin, and ticarcillin/clavulanate. As a result there was a significant decrease not only in the resistant acinetobacter but also in resistance to other antibiotics.[14] There was no adverse effect on mortality, hospital or ICU stay nor any delay in appropriate antibiotics being given, despite the restrictive policy. Infection control procedures did not alter during the period of the study. It was concluded antibiotic use should be controlled and that the exact controls should reflect those which are optimal for a particular healthcare system.

Over the past 30 years the literature has been full of anecdotes supporting the concept that cycling through the different classes of antibiotic is able to control antibiotic resistance, although there is no long-term evidence available. We should be cautious of extrapolating from short-term studies, such as the study from Iceland[11] addressing the problem of resistant pneumococci in the community where reduction in antibiotic prescribing lead to decrease in the rate of incidence of resistant pneumococci. It is known that in the community, multiresistant clones can come and go with a natural cycle of an epidemic, even without altered antibiotic prescribing, such that it may just be pure chance that resistance patterns change. Certainly in the community it is much more difficult to influence antibiotic resistance. In a hospital and particularly in the ICU the rapid flux of patients means that resistance clones are diluted. During the 1970s there were major aminoglycoside resistance problems in the USA with resistant rates to gentamicin and tobramycin of about 40%. Using active measures, after 2 years resistance problems were less, despite a return to gentamicin. Such studies are very poorly controlled observational studies, but they are part of the history of what might become a successful strategy of antibiotic cycling or antibiotic rotation. At the moment good trials are lacking.

Conclusion

It is almost certain that there is a causative association between antibiotic use and the development of resistance. Given the recent worldwide escalation in resistance and the overwhelming evidence of unnecessary antibiotic use, the sensible approach to the control of antibiotic resistance is to control antibiotic use. The important question is how, rather than whether, but much research is still needed. It is probably the case that limiting antibiotic prescribing, and not conscious antibiotic cycling, is the way forward.

References

1 Kunin CM. Antibiotic armageddon. *Clin Infect Dis* 1997; **25**:240–1.
2 Gould IM, Hampson J, Taylor EW, Wood MJ. Hospital antibiotic control measures in the UK. *J Antimicrob Chemother* 1994; **34**:21–42.
3 Bergogne-Berezin E. Interaction between antibiotics, bacteria and the human immune system: the clinical relevance of *in vitro* testing. *J Chemother* 1997; **9**:109–15.

4 McGowan JE, Tenover FC. Control of antimicrobial resistance in the health care system. *Infect Dis Clin North Am* 1997; **11**:297–311.
5 Schrag SJ, Perrot V, Levin BR. Adaptation to the fitness costs of antibiotic resistance in *Escherichia coli*. *Proc R Soc Med Series B* 1997; **264**:1287–91.
6 Amyes SGB, Gould IM. Trimethoprim resistance plasmids. *Ann Microbiol* 1984; **135B**:177–86.
7 Nikaido H. Multidrug efflux pumps of gram negative bacteria. *J Bacteriol* 1996; **178**:5853–9.
8 Gould IM. Risk factors for acquisition of multiply drug resistant gram negative bacteria. *Eur J Clin Microbiol Infect Dis* 1994; **13**:S30–8.
9 Lipsitch M, Levine BR. The population dynamics of antimicrobial chemotherapy. *Antimicrob Agents Chemother* 1997; **41**:363–73.
10 Gerding DN, Larson TA, Hughes RA, Weiler M, Shanholtzer C, Peterson LR. Aminoglycoside resistance and aminoglycoside usage. *Antimicrob Agents Chemother* 1991; **35**:1284–90.
11 Arason VA, Kristinsson KG, Sigurdsson JA, Stephansdottir G, Molstad S, Gudmundsson S. Do antimicrobials increase the carriage rate of penicillin resistant pneumococci in children? *Br Med J* 1996; **313**:387–91.
12 Seppala H, Klaukka T, Vuopio-Varkila J, *et al.* The effect of changes in the consumption of macrolide antibiotics on erythromycin resistance in group A streptococci in Finland. *N Engl J Med* 1997; **7**:441–6.
13 Aubry-Damon H, Legrand P, Brun-Buisson C, Astier A, Soussy CJ, Leciercq R. Re-emergence of gentamicin-susceptible strains of methicillin-resistant *Staphylococcus aureus:* roles of an infection control program and changes in aminoglycoside use. *Clin Infect Dis* 1997; **25**:647–53.
14 Gould IM. A review of the role of antibiotic policies in the control of antibiotic resistance. *J Antimicrob Chemother* 1999; **43**:459–65.

7: Antibiotic policies in the intensive care unit

VANYA GANT

Introduction

All antibiotics alter normal bacterial flora, and select for natural and acquired antibiotic resistance with subsequent dissemination through initially asymptomatic colonisation and cross-infection. Resistance to antibiotics compromises therapy, and policies or guidelines for antibiotic prescribing may help to rationalise and reduce antibiotic usage, resulting in a reduction in costs and delaying the emergence of resistance. This article will address issues relating to proscriptive antibiotic policies on the intensive care unit (ICU).

Setting the scene

Patients on the ICU are at a higher risk of hospital-acquired infection than other hospitalised patients, and are subjected to invasive procedures facilitating the entry of micro-organisms. Outcome is dependent not only on the severity of the underlying condition but also on the vulnerability of the patients to infection. Accordingly the acquisition of antibiotic resistance has marked implications for treatment options in the infected ICU patient. Antibiotic resistance varies in both type and extent between ICUs and the rational choice of antibiotic has to reflect resistance patterns in individual units. Procedures must be in place to assess the prevalence of potentially pathogenic organisms, which should be used to design pathogenic organisms and local treatment strategies.[1]

Limiting antibiotic prescribing

It is clear that the emergence of resistance is linked to increased antibiotic usage. Adequate infection control strategies should reduce the need for antibiotic prescribing and hence decrease the selective pressure for the emergence of resistant organisms. Effective infection control practices are addressed thoroughly in Chapter 2. There is still some controversy as to whether narrow- or broad-spectrum empirical therapy is more appropriate, although the anxiety generated by treating (possibly ineffectively) unknown infection with narrow-spectrum antibiotics usually pushes clinicians towards broad-spectrum antibiotics, at least until a causative organism is found. Whilst this broad-spectrum approach has prompted comments about the need for, and value of, blood cultures because common blood culture isolates allegedly have sensitivities to antimicrobials which can be reliably predicted,[2] Cunney *et al.* suggest that in practice this is not the case.[3] Thus, 24% of patients who received empirical treatment were later found to have an isolate which was either resistant or only moderately sensitive to the antibiotic regimen used.

Why does inappropriate prescribing occur?

There are a number of reasons why doctors might prescribe antibiotics in ways considered inappropriate by microbiologists, either in terms of what or how. Probably the most important driver for non-evidence based and possibly irrational prescribing in the context of critical illness is the "septic slump", which represents a final pathological common pathway prompted by many causes. It takes courage and determination not to treat increasing cooling requirements, inotrope dosage and inhaled oxygen fraction with easily prescribed broad-spectrum antibiotics. It is unfortunately a fact of life that many, if not the majority, of these patients may be "slumping" for a reason other than an antibiotic responsive one. Unfortunately we simply do not have the rapid technology to better define the reason for clinical deterioration in the setting of the "septic slump" – this is because we don't understand it well enough yet. Other causes include inadequate knowledge of the probable nature and aetiology of the infection, inadequate knowledge of the nature and efficacy of antibiotics, or both. Fear of litigation as a result of delay or failure to cover every possibility may also direct prescribing.

Antibiotic policies

Rational prescribing in this context implies a knowledge of the chosen drug pharmacokinetics and toxicity profile, knowledge of probable causative agents and their susceptibility to antimicrobial agents, and clinical endpoints of efficacy once prescribed. All ICUs should embrace some form of antibiotic policy to rationalise prescribing. It is important to define the terms of reference for the policy: its aims should be clearly stated, and these might incorporate several practical goals which can be worked towards (Box 7.1). It is important that clinicians retain their clinical freedom and are not made to feel either devalued or restricted, in order that they can on the one hand appropriately assess and respond to the needs of individual patients and circumstances, and on the other feel empowered and comfortable with decisions which are in line with policy. The guidelines for antibiotic use embedded in such policy represent an active approach to the control of antibiotic use, by offering expert and evidence based guidance on optimal therapy for specific infections tuned for local circumstances. The group devising such guidelines should ideally include an intensivist, a surgeon, a microbiologist, and a pharmacist.

Box 7.1 Aims of antibiotic prescribing policies

- To provide the most effective treatment
- To advise and educate on rational prescribing – e.g. duplication/spectrum of action/sensitivity
- To limit the use of prophylactic prescribing of antibiotics
- To delay or prevent emergence of resistant strains
- To limit cost
- To minimise adverse events

The format of such formal written guidelines is vital. The policy should be short, readable, and regularly updated. However it is important that the guidelines are not superficial and offer comprehensive advice. A well written and "marketed" policy should not preclude the ability to respond to specific needs of patient care, but should reduce, for example, the use of inappropriate combinations of antibiotics, frankly unnecessary antibiotic prescription, and surgical prophylaxis extending beyond the operating theatre.

Over 60% of patients on an ICU are receiving antibiotics at any one time; much of this usage is questionable if not completely inappropriate. The triggers for antibiotic prescription in the ICU are, however, steeped in tradition, and any change will be potentially painful for clinicians when such crystallised prescribing habits are challenged. There are various non-confrontational tactics which can be used to restrict antibiotic overprescribing. These might include restricting the antibiotics available in pharmacy, monitoring of requests for new antibiotics, and provision of objective information on new drugs before clinicians are approached by pharmaceutical representatives. The economics of antibiotic development not unreasonably forces industry to work hard at persuading clinicians to move over to prescribing new wonder drugs. Furthermore they are sometimes aided and abetted by microbiologists publicly extolling the imminent arrival of the "doomsday superbug". In this context it should be noted that it currently costs about £600 million to take an antibiotic through clinical trials to the marketplace. It is therefore perfectly reasonable for a pharmaceutical company to market towards sales and profits beyond this figure – which is formidable when one considers the relatively small market that ICUs represent in the grander scheme of things. It may even be that industry will no longer consider this particular market attractive, potentially leaving doctors and their patients without the tools for therapy.

Do antibiotic-prescribing policies work?

The only way to answer this question for individual units is through audit, and a number of questions which might be asked can easily be identified (Box 7.2). Several studies have shown that antibiotic-prescribing guidelines do help. One of the first such studies[4] reported the change in antibiotic-prescribing practice after a "quality of use" audit, where antibiotic prescribing was defined as rational (choice and dosage appropriate for the infection, whether proven or suspected, or appropriate for prophylaxis), questionable (insufficient clinical or microbiological data to enable classification), or irrational (no indication whatsoever for the use of antibiotics). Feedback to prescribers resulted in significant changes in prescribing habits, particularly with regard to surgical prophylaxis; presumably because most of this is built on appropriately constructed trials from which a good evidence base has developed.

Box 7.2 Suggested audit areas for evaluating impact of antibiotic policies

- Site of infection
- Clinical, radiological, microbiological evidence for infection
- Suspected organism
- Organism(s) actually isolated
- Appropriateness of prescribing an antibiotic at all
- Appropriateness of actual antibiotic regimen used – dose, duration, regimen

---

The method of evaluation of the impact of antibiotic policies should be planned at the outset, and agreed between those involved. The type of evaluation used must be dependent on local resources but must be specific, simple, and meaningful. More importantly, the findings should be shared and acted upon.[5] Audit of antibiotic use should not be seen as either a threat to clinicians or as an attempt at policing their antibiotic-prescribing choices. It should be a means of justifying the selection of antibiotics as a result of critical analysis, resulting in altered prescribing patterns and reduced costs.[6]

Saving money was achieved in a French ICU following implementation of an agreed rational antibiotic prescribing policy for 2 years.[7] However, although antibiotic use and hence cost was cut by 19% in year 1 and 22% in year 2, the nosocomial infection rate was not altered. In a much earlier study of a urological ward, a policy to restrict antibiotic sensitivity reports resulted in better compliance with prescribing guidelines since antibiotics for which sensitivity data were not provided were rarely prescibed.[8] Recently outbreaks of *Clostridium difficile* in Medicine for the Elderly Units in two UK hospitals were controlled effectively through combinations of very restrictive antibiotic-prescribing guidelines and improved infection control strategies, and resulted in a considerable reduction in costs.[9,10]

Antibiotic resistance is increasing through increased antibiotic usage, whether such use is rational or irrational. It has been suggested that the limitation of use of such drugs where resistance is high may result in reversion to more sensitive states. In 1970, the incidence of erythromycin-resistant *Staphylococcus aureus* was decreased when erythromycin prescribing was heavily restricted, but re-emerged when it was re-introduced.[11] Resistance mechanisms are complex and withdrawal of a single antibiotic may be insufficient to limit resistance.[12] Indeed, also in 1970, withdrawal of all antibiotics was implemented in a neurosurgical unit which successfully limited a fatal outbreak of *Klebsiella aerogenes*.[13] The study was all the more interesting because no deaths could be attributed to lack of antibiotics during the study period. In 1998 however, ceftazidime restriction policies in an attempt to decrease colonisation with ceftazidime-resistant gram-negative bacilli in a paediatric ICU in the USA were unsuccessful, since although ceftazidime use was curtailed by 96%, the number of resistant organisms increased.[14] There are many reasons for such findings, such as the pressure put upon the unit by the hospital's bacterial ecology as a whole, and the genetic stability of the antibiotic resistance elements within the bacterial population to name but two. Certainly restriction of ceftazidime usage seems to have been effective in preventing the development and acquisition of vancomycin-resistant enterococci (VRE) amongst patients in a busy haematology unit.[15]

Failure of antibiotic policies

Implementation of policy guidelines may fail, primarily due to lack of communication. A restrictive policy requiring consultant signature for all prescribing will be met with dismay if not disdain by both consultant and junior staff alike. Microbiologists need to be available for advice but a requirement for approval of all prescribing is unworkable. Those defining antibiotic guidelines must not be seen as misguided, confused or, worse still, obstructive.

Conclusion

The approach to limitation of emergence of resistance should be multi-faceted, through reduced and more appropriate antibiotic prescribing and adequate infection control. What antibiotics are used should be used appropriately in the right doses; newer agents such as linezolid or sitafloxacin should be kept firmly in the cupboard in order that they can be relied on in those moments where nothing else will do. Possibly the best solution for the ICU is the daily attendance by a clinically oriented microbiologist with a positive and communicative attitude, and a pen for crossing off all those unneccessary antibiotics.

References

1 Tullu MS, Deshmukh CT, Baveja SM. Bacterial profile and antimicrobial susceptibility patterns in catheter related nosocomial infections. *J Postgrad Med* 1998; **44**:7–13.
2 Greenwood D. Antimicrobial susceptibility testing: are we wasting our time? *Br J Biomed Sci* 1993; **50**:31–4.
3 Cunney RJ, McNamara EB, Alansari N, Loo B, Smyth EG. The impact of blood culture reporting and clinical liaison on the empiric treatment of bacteraemia. *J Clin Pathol* 1997; **50**:1010–12.
4 Achong MR, Wood J, Theal HK, Goldberg R, Thompson DA. Changes in hospital antibiotic therapy after a quality of use study. *Lancet* 1977; **ii**:1118–22.
5 Nathwani D. How do you measure the impact of an antibiotic policy? *J Hosp Infect* 1999; **43**:S265–8.
6 Gould IM. Stewardship of antibiotic use and resistance surveillance: the international scene. *J Hosp Infect* 1999; **43**:S253–60.
7 Blanc P, Von Elm BE, Geissler A, *et al*. Economic impact of a rational use of antibiotics in intensive care. *Intensive Care Med* 1999; **25**:1407–12.
8 Casewell MW, Pugh S, Dalton MT. Correlation of antibiotic usage with an antibiotic policy in a urological ward. *J Hosp Infect* 1981; **2**:55–61.
9 McNulty C, Logan M , Donald IP, *et al*. Successful control of a *Clostridium difficile* infection in an elderly care unit through use of a restrictive policy. *J Antimicrob Chemother* 1977; **40**:707–11.
10 Ludlam H, Brown N, Sule O, Redpath C, Coni N, Owen G. An antibiotic policy associated with reduced risk of *Clostridium difficile*-associated diarrhoea. *Age Ageing* 1999; **28**:578–80.
11 Ridley M, Barrie D, Lynn R, Stead KC. Antibiotic resistant *Staphylococcus aureus* and hospital antibiotic policies. *Lancet* 1970; **i**:230–3.

12 Lowbury EJL, Babb JR, Roe E. Clearance from a hospital of Gram negative bacilli that transfer carbenicillin resistance to *Pseudomonas aeruginosa*. *Lancet* 1972; **ii**:941–5.

13 Price DJE, Sleigh JD. Control of infection due to *Klebsiella aerogenes* in a neurosurgical unit by withdrawal of all antibiotics. *Lancet* 1970; **ii**:1213–15.

14 Toltzis P, Yamashita T, Vilt L, *et al*. Antibiotic restriction does not alter endemic colonization with resistant gram negative rods in a pediatric intensive care unit. *Crit Care Med* 1998; **26**:1893–9.

15 Bradley SJ, Wilson AL, Allen MA, *et al*. The control of hyperendemic glycopeptide-resistant *Enterococcus* spp. on a haematology unit by changing antibiotic usage. *J Antimicrob Chemother* 1999; **43**:261–6.